CHINESE MEDICINE 101:
START WITH THE FOUNDATIONS

Part one of a two-part journey into understanding Chinese Medicine

By Cat Calhoun, MAcOm, L.Ac.

Cats TCM Notes Press
San Miguel de Allende, Mexico

This page intentionally left blank

*For DeLora, my sunshine and my rest.
Thank you with all my heart for your supporting
and for sticking with me through Chinese Medicine School!*

This page intentionally left blank

ACKNOWLEDGMENTS

No one does anything truly on their own. I thought myself totally self-sufficient before I dove into the study of Chinese medicine. When that journey began, my eyes opened to the myriads of those who were actively helping me, those who have gone before, and even those who will come long after I'm gone. We are interconnected. You are me, I am you.

I especially want to thank Dr. Qianzhi Wu, my teacher and one of the wisest souls I have ever encountered. Thank you for your wisdom and your teaching, for your patience and guidance, for the gift of Qigong which I would not have seen with the beauty that it is without you showing it to me.

Thank you to Master Junfeng Li, my Shengzhen Qigong teacher. Qigong kept me sane and healthy in school and for this I thank you.

Thank you to Lisa Lapwing, a most awesome practitioner based in Orlando Florida. We studied together, practiced together, we practiced *on* each other in student clinic, and then we became each others' practitioners! Not having Lisa in my daily life is my one giant regret about moving to Mexico.

Thank you to my buds: Donna "Needles" Tatum, Tiffany Chiu Peralez, Vanessa Olsen, Andi Kohn, Mark Hernandez, and Katherine Webster. To Georgie Hoiseth, a kick ass practitioner and fellow computer geek, I thank thee! To Rita Ramirez, I would *NOT* want to be on this journey without you!

And to so may more who have loved, supported, and believed in me, I express my gratitude and thanks. May the deity of your choice look favorably upon you all!

Cat Calhoun

This page intentionally left blank

CHAPTER 1:
The History of Chinese Medicine

Chinese civilization has existed in written record for about 5000 years; Chinese medicine for about 4500 years. **The Yellow Emperor** is the legendary ancestor the Chinese civilization and is an important figure not only in Chinese culture, but in the spiritual system of Daoism. Said to have been born in 2704 BC, and to have become emperor in 2697 BC, he is often credited with the invention of wooden houses and carts, boats, the bow and arrow, and the early system of Chinese writing. Some tales credit him with the invention of coins as money and with the Chinese systems of government. He is seen as a very wise man whose reign was a golden age in China. When he died, he was said to have become an Immortal.

HUANG DI NEI JING

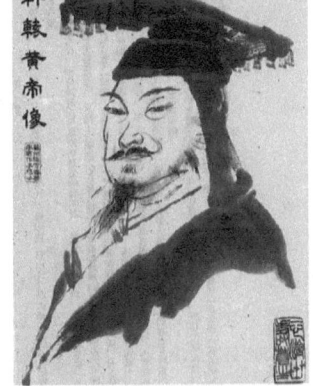

The *Yellow Emperor's Internal* Classics or the *Huang Di Nei Jing,* is the most important book in Chinese medicine. Attributed to Huang Di, or the Yellow Emperor, this book lays out the foundations and fundamentals of the discipline and practices of Chinese medicine.

The *Huang Di Nei Jing,* though attributed to the famed Yellow Emperor, is actually a compilation of the works of many herbalists over several decades, spanning the Spring and Autumn period of Chinese history (770 – 476 BC) to the Warring states period (475 – 221 BC)

> Cat's Note: You'll be studying this book in several classes during your education. Advanced Needling and Herbal Classics both rely heavily on the book.

The *Huang Di Nei Jing* is divided into 2 parts:

- *Su* Wen or *Plain/Simple Questions* - the fundamentals of Chinese medicine
- *Ling Shu* or *Miraculous/Spiritual Pivot* which details the channels, point locations, etc.

HUA TUO

Hua Tuo (AD 110-207) is the first famous surgeon in Chinese medicine. The first recorded development and use of anesthesia is credited to Hua Tuo and he is famously known for his vast knowledge of human anatomy. Hua Tuo preferred simple methods of acupuncture and herbs, using a small number of acupuncture points in his treatments and formulas with only a few herbs. As an illustrative from Dr. Qianzhi Wu's notes:

> One day a patient came to see Hua Tuo. Hua Tuo diagnosed the patient with ulcerative colitis (bleeding ulcer in the large intestine). He decided that surgery was needed. He gave the patient "anesthetic powder." When the patient lost feeling, he cut the abdomen, located the ulcer in the intestine and (probably) resected the bowel. After sewing the patient back together he applied "Spirits Lotion." One month later the patient was completely recovered.

Hua Tuo practiced Qigong and invented/taught a style called Frolic of the Five Animals or Five Animal Qigong, which is still practiced today. Five Animal Qigong is based on the movements and behaviors of the Tiger, Deer, Bear, Ape, and Crane. It is a powerful technique for cancer patients, as cancer cells tend to shrink and recede with regular practice of this qigong.

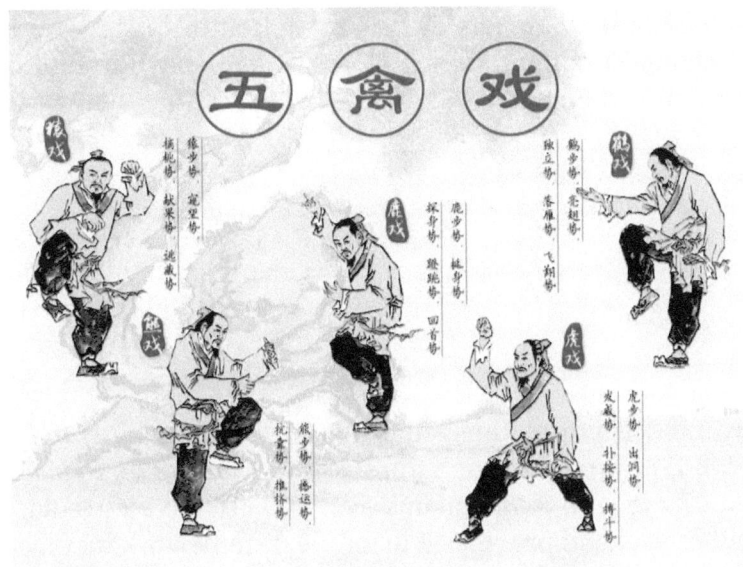

Hua Tuo invented the Jiaji points, 34 bilateral points along the erector spinae muscles of the back, which interact with the *central* nervous system, and *can* therefore help some paraplegics and quadriplegic patients regain function in certain circumstances. All other acu-points treat at the level of the peripheral nervous system, but these points have an effect on the gap junction between the central and peripheral nervous endings.

Hua Tuo died at the age of 97, not from old age, but because a general named Zao Cao ordered his death. Zao Cao had contracted an illness called "Tou Feng" or head wind. The general came to see Hua Tuo and was advised to have an operation. Suspecting Hua Tuo wanted to harm him, the general had him executed.

ZHANG ZHONGJING

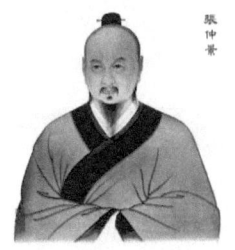

Zhang ZhongJing (also called Zhang Ji – AD 412-220), the most famous of China's ancient herbal doctors, was originally a provincial governor who resigned his position in order to pursue the study and practice of medicine. When he was approximately 50 years old a deadly plague swept through China. Over 2/3 of Zhang

Zhongjing's family members died as a result of this plague. With sadness, Zhang Zhongjing decided to dedicate himself to finding a solution to this problem.

> Cat's Note: A febrile disease is a communicable disease. When Zhang Zhongjing was alive the predominant communicable diseases began with symptoms of cold. That's why you will see diseases in Zhang Zhongjing's works referred to as "Cold Injured Diseases" – because it was cold that injured the body first.

After several decades he finished his work, titled *Shang Han Lun* or *Shang Han Za Bing Lun* which translates to *Treatise on Febrile Diseases*. *Shang Han Lun* contains over 100 effective formulas, many still in use, and provides a theoretical framework that led to hundreds of books analyzing, explaining, and refining his theories. It contains 397 articles and 112 prescriptions and is considered to be a cornerstone in TCM history.

Another section of the *Shang Han Lun* is well known for some of the herbal treatment formulas it contains, many of which are still commonly used in clinic. The gynecological remedy Xiao Yao San (also known as Tang-Kuei and Peony Formula, Dang Gui Xiao Yao San, and "Free and Easy Wanderer") is still used for infertility, disorders during pregnancy, prevention of miscarriage, post-partum weakness, irregular periods, painful periods, menstrual dysfunction, and PMS syndromes.

This great work could have been lost to history, but for the efforts of Wang ShuHe. Wang ShuHe recovered the book, reworked it a bit and split it into 2 parts. *The Treatise on Febrile Diseases* (*Shang Han Lun*) is the part which discusses the invasion of the body by externally introduced pathogens. The second part, *The Golden Chamber* (aka, *Jing Kui Yao Lue*) covers internal disease, diet, stress, etc.

HUANGFU MI

Huangfu Mi (214-282 AD) lived to see the end of the later Han Dynasty. He is famous for his skills in acupuncture therapy. He composed many literary works and was very influential during his time. He studied Chinese medicine carefully and by the end of his life had compiled one of the prominent acupuncture works in history, *Huang Di Zhenjiu Jia Yi Jing* or (in English) *The Yellow Emperors Acupuncture A and B*.

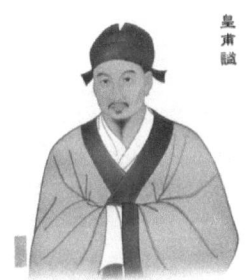

This classic, often nicknamed *Jia Yi Jing*, consists of 12 scrolls and 128 chapters. It not only summarized the entire body of knowledge about acupuncture at the time, but added a sizeable amount of new information. Later generations of acupuncturists needed only to learn Huangfu Mi's book to understand the secrets of the art. This classic influenced the art of acupuncture in China as well as countries around the world such as France, Korea, and Japan.

WANG SHUHE

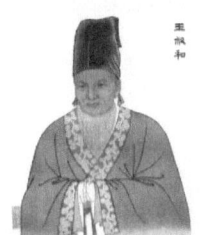

Wang Shuhe, who you might remember from the discussion about Zhang Zhongjing above, lived from AD 210 – 285, during the Western Jin dynasty and is the great pulse diagnosis expert in Chinese medical history. He wrote *Mai Jing* or *The Pulse Classics* (which you might also see titled "The Classic of Pulses") detailing 24 pulses. The 10 scrolls of this work describe the pulse positions and methods for reading the pulse. We use this as the basis for our current pulse diagnosis, though we now learn 28 different pulses in our basic education.

SUN SIMIAO

Sun Simiao is the "King of Herbs." Sun Simiao (AD 590-682) was a famous doctor during the Tang dynasty. Sun Simiao is famous not only for his herbal knowledge, but also for his medical ethics and desire to help the poor.

He may be the first guy in recorded history to practice the community acupuncture model, charging fees on a sliding scale and recommending food therapy as a simple remedy to illness. He recommended seaweed to people living in the mountains who suffered from goiter and recommended the liver of oxen and sheep for people suffering from night blindness. (Later you will learn that the Liver "opens" to the eyes. When the energy of the Liver is out of balance, it can result in eye problems, among other things.)

A Daoist master, Sun Simiao understood the virtue, spirit, and energy of plant medicines. "Human life is worth a thousand gold bars, with a virtue of one prescription you can fix it" is a quote from Sun Simiao. In 652 he compiled the famous *Qian Jin Yi Fang*, also called *Prescriptions Worth a Thousand Gold for Emergencies*, 30 scrolls worth of herbal scripts. Later he composed a second work of 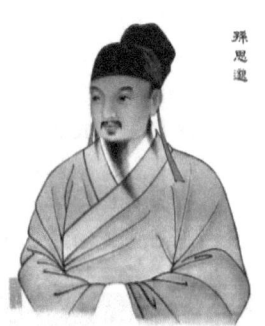 30 scrolls, a continuation of his herbal philosophy and prescriptions. He also sought demon-dispelling remedies, including spells, herbal formulas and toxic alchemical preparations.

> Cat Note: This is some of the energetic and magical aspect of Chinese Medicine that gets somewhat swept under the rug in western TCM schools, as it is not considered an 'acceptable' form of healing to the western biomedicine 'machine' that it is so popular to fit into now. Try not to discount this doaist shaman just because his wording doesn't 'fit' into our current culture.

Liu Wansu

Liu Wansu (1120-1200) lived during the Jing Dynasty. He observed the high incidence of fever and inflammation in serious disease and noted that febrile disease seemed to be more warm-focused ("warm injured") than cold-focused ("cold inured") in his time period. Contemporary and previous practitioners,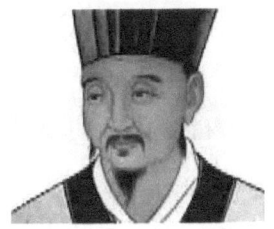
since the time of Zhang Zhongjing had focused on the idea of "cold injured" illnesses, so disease was often treated with herbs that warmed the body.

Noting the heat signs predominant in the early stages of diseases of his time, and that warming herbs seemed to be making problems worse, he promoted the idea of using *cool* natured herbs to treat and balance febrile conditions that had symptoms and signs of too much heat in the body. Though this was a thought that was counter to mainstream, his writings nevertheless heavily influenced the later concept of *"wen bing"* or epidemic febrile diseases, which corresponded to and yet pre-dated the western idea of contagious diseases.

Liu Wansu also undertook a detailed study of the *Nei Jing Su Wen* or *Plain Questions of the Yellow Emperor's Internal Classic*, describing the etiology (origin or cause) of disease in relation to the teachings of this famous text.

Zhang Zihe

Zhang Zihe (1156-1228AD) is known as the developer of the 'Attacking School' of Chinese medicine. This philosophy emphasized the use of diaphoretics, emetics, and purgatives to attack pathogens and drive them out of the body. (This is a revival of the early Han Dynasty techniques of driving out demons.)

Pathogens are seen as an excess in Chinese medicine and these techniques eliminate that excess by dispelling or removing them.

You will often see this referred to as "sedating" the excess, which is a kind way of saying you're going to kick it to the curb. "Sedate excesses, tonify deficiencies" is a common theme in Chinese medicine.

LI DONGYUAN (AKA LI GAO)

Li Dongyuan (Li Gao) lived from 1180 - 1252 AD and is best known for his philosophy that most diseases were due to injury to the Stomach/Spleen system as the result of intemperance in eating and drinking, overwork, and the seven emotions. This philosophy is still employed: an overuse of cold and sedative herbs, foods, or medications lead to disease and obesity.

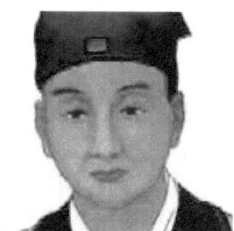

Li Gao said that good digestion is the key to good health. Indeed this has borne out in recent studies which concluded that 80% of the immune system lives in the gut. Li Gao detailed this philosophy, practice, and many of his herbal scripts (which are still widely used in TCM practice today) in *Pi Wei Lun* or *Treatise on the Stomach and Spleen*. One of his famous scripts and one of the most used is Bu Zhong Yi Qi Tang (ginseng and astragalus) which treats muscle atrophy, prolapse of internal organs, fatigue, and fibromyalgia as well as boosting immunity.

ZHU DANXI

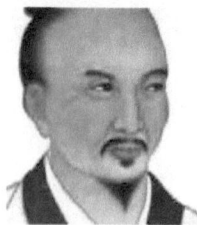

Zhu Danxi is also known as Zhu Zhenheng (1280-1358AD). He believed that people suffered from chronic disease mainly due to overindulgences in pleasurable foods, drink, and activities which led to an eventual debility of the Yin Essence in the body. He recommended temperance in all things and the use of tonic formulas, especially those nourishing the Kidney and Liver.

Dr. Qianzhi Wu, one of my professors and a truly amazing doctor, says 80-85% of disease is lifestyle related, including high blood pressure, high blood sugar, and high cholesterol. This results from

Yin deficiency/Yang excess. To nourish Yin, nourish the Kidney and Liver while reducing your desires. Yin is the body's essence, fluids and blood. Yang is activity, mental effort, and thinking. You need daylight to produce Yang and night to nourish the Yin. Too little sleep results in a lack of Yin -- so don't work the night shift if you can avoid it! To remedy an excess of Yang and a deficiency of Yin, get to sleep earlier, reduce your desires and practice temperance in all things. This is the 'middle way' of Buddhism. Qigong and meditation can help with the desire and temperance thang.

ZHANG JINGUYE

Zhang Jingyue lived from 1583 – 1640 A.D. during the Ming Dynasty. He was a prolific writer and produced works on pulse diagnosis, gynecology, pediatrics, surgery, and an analysis of the *Nei Jing* which is referred to in Chinese medicine circles as the *Lei Jing*.

He said Yang Qi and Yin Essence are rooted in the Kidney. He therefore advocated that life cultivation should concentrate on enhancing the Kidney with simultaneous consideration of Yin and Yang. He also established a set of tonic prescriptions with the actions of mutual tonification of Yin and Yang which are still in use. In addition, he also put forward the theory of "life cultivation in the middle-aged" (which attaches importance to life cultivation in middle-aged people). This has a positive significance for prevention of premature aging and senile diseases.

LI SHIZHEN

Li Shizhen lived from 1518 – 1593. He is considered to be China's greatest naturalist. He was very interested in the proper classification of the components of nature. He sifted through the vast array of herbal lore over a span of 40 years and wrote his information into the *Ben Cao Gang Mu* (or in English, *The Copendium of Materia Medica*), a treatise on pharmacopoeia, botany, zoology, mineralogy and metallurgy.

This book has been reprinted frequently and five of the originals still exist. (There's even an app called *Ben Cao* for your mobile devices. Good stuff. I recommend it.) A rough translation of the herbal entries was published in English by two British doctors who were working in China at the end of the 19th century (Porter and Smith). Exerpts of it were published in Europe since 1656 as well. *Ben Cao Gang Mu* contains 1,892 different herbs, is divided into 6 sections, 52 scrolls and 60 different categories.

> For some historical perspective, during this same time period (around 1550 AD), the Jesuits were formed, the Spanish had recently finished killing off the Aztec empire, Nostradamus wrote his first almanac, and Altan Khan besieged Peking/Bejing (there's a PBS video about this regarding the Great Wall of China and how Altan Khan broke through it and torched the 'burbs of Peking).

WU YOUXING

Wu Youxing lived from 1582 to 1652 AD. He developed the concept that some diseases were caused by transmissible agents, which he called pestilential factors or "liqi." His book, *Wen Yi Lun* or *Treatise on Acute Epidemic Febrile Diseases* is regarded as the main etiological work that introduced the concept of germs causing epidemic disease. Ultimately, this was attributed to Westerners... of course.

Until Wu Youxing, disease was thought to be caused by one or a combination of the six evils: Wind, Cold, Damp, Heat, Summer Heat, and Dryness. Wu Youxing's work did not *negate* or disprove the influence of these six evils, but rather added the 7th one in the list: *Liqi* or transmissible agents.

> Sidebar:
> - Infectious diseases due to viral infection (mumps, strep, HIV, SARS, Bird flu, etc.) are considered to be *warm* or warm-injured diseases.
> - Autoimmune diseases come from *inside* the individual, not from outside sources like febrile disease. These are due to an imbalance of Yin and Yang.

YE TIANSHI

Ye Tianshi (AD 1690-1760) is famous for his thesis on febrile diseases, *Wen Re Lun* or *Treatise on Epidemic Fevers,* published in 1746. He postulated the transmission of disease in four stages, with the first stage affecting the body first and progressing further inward as follows:

- **Wei level**
  The affect is on the exterior limits of the body.

- **Qi level**
  Getting deeper, but still fairly exterior by comparison to the next stages.

- **Jing or Nutritive level**
  This is deeper penetration into the body's defenses. By the time a disease gets this far it has gotten to the storehouse of the body and is difficult to stop because now it has resources to nourish it. Kind of like enemy troops capturing a supply line, you know?

- **Xue or Blood level**
  This is the deepest level. Now the patient is in deep, deep trouble. No good can come from this! The prognosis for this patient is not good.

Ye Tianshi also wrote a book, even more famous than the last, called *Detailed Analysis of Febrile Diseases* or *Wen Bing Tiao Bian.*

You'll study these Four Stages later in Diagnostics and will often hear it refered to as simply *Wen Bing*.

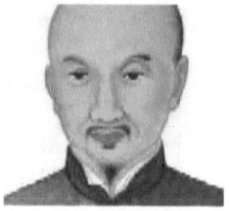

If you take the time to trace the history of disease, you might see that most diseases, 2000-5000 years ago were mostly cold injured diseases (disease that begin with a lot of cold signs in the body) and were treated with warm and hot herbs to counter what was seen as the cold nature of the invading disease.

Liu Wansu was on the cutting edge of the shift in disease, noticing that diseases were becoming hot in nature and should be treated with cooling herbs. This is still applicable today, though it takes an astute doctor knowledgeable and competent in Chinese medicine diagnostics to be able to tell the difference between the two.

THE BIG TAKEAWAY

Though I cannot predict what your particular professors will emphasize on tests, the important takeaways here are:

Four Great Classics of Oriental Medicine

> Know the names of these books and who wrote each
> 1. Yellow Emperor's Internal Classic – *Huang Di Neijing*
> 2. Treatise on Febrile Diseases – *Shang Han Lun*
> 3. Golden Chamber - *Jing Kui Yao Lue*
> 4. Detailed Analysis of Febrile Diseases - *Wen Bing Tiao Bian*

Four Great Doctors in the Jing Dynasty

> Know their names and contributions to Chinese medicine
> 1. Liu Wansu – cold herbs for hot diseases
> 2. Zhang Zihe – the "Attacking School"
> 3. Li Dongyuan – *Treatise on Stomach and Spleen*
> 4. Zhu Danxi – disease comes from overindulgence

Chapter 2
Yin Yang Theory

YIN YANG THEORY

4000-5000 years ago China was predomiantly agricultural. The sun was the primary source of energy and sunlight (or the lack thereof) was used to measure time, which had special meaning for a society centered on growing crops.

The Origins of Yin and Yang

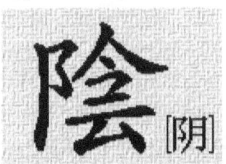

The glyph for *yin*, shown to the left consists of several other distinct characters or glyphs. The first is a hill, the B looking portion to the left. To the right of this is the character for the word *today*. Below this is the character meaning *cloudy*. If it's cloudy when you're observing the sky, then it is a Yin day, as you cannot see the sun and sunlight represents yang.

Yang, as previously stated, has a lot to do with sunlight. To the right is the glyph that means *yang* in Chinese. Note the same hill on the graphic. The top portion of the glyph represents the sun rising. A person standing on this "hill" looking at the sky sees sunshine when the sky isn't cloudy at sunrise. The bottom part of the glyph represents rays of sunlight. Sunny days are yang days.

So as you can tell the origin of yin and yang has to do with observing the day and the sun and the season.

The Measurement of Yin and Yang

Some days are more Yang in nature than other days. Winter sun, for instance, is different than summer sun. You can measure the volume and degree of Yang. In China, measurement of the shadows determined yin (shadow) and

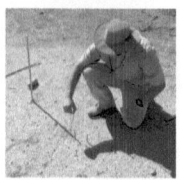 Yang (sunlight). At high noon a pole held vertically casts no shadow, so this is considered to be a time of full Yang.

Eventually this was depicted in a sort of stylized shorthand as a long unbroken line like this, called the Yang Xiao: _____.

Yin which is shadow was drawn as a broken line, representing both the shadow and the pole: _____ _____
This is the Yin Xiao. Combinations of these stylized symbols represented different times of day.

____ ____ _____	Sun rising. Yang is coming up from below and yin is receding. This also represents the concept of Spring with the yang growing upward.
_____ _____	Noon or Midday. Yang is full now. Two yang xiao represent this. This also represents the Summer season when yang is strongest.
_____ ____ ____	Sun setting. Yin is coming and Yang is receding. This also represents fall or Autumn when Yin is overtaking Yang.
____ ____ ____ ____	Midnight. Yin is full. Two Yin Xiao represent this. This also represents the Winter season when Yin is the strongest.

The Ba Gua or Trigram

Additional lines were added beyond the yin xiao and yang xiao at some point in time. The result is the following:

Qian	Kun	Li	Kan
Heaven	Earth	Fire (you need the yin of wood to get fire)	Water

Zhan	Gen	Xun	Dui
Thunder	Mountain	Wind	Marsh or Lake

The Hexagram

Combination of 2 of the tri-grams above to give 64 hexagrams. This version of yin/yang measurement is contained in the *I Ching, The Book of Changes*. The source of this change is the sun. Winter is the time when the energy has receded downward. In Summer the energy is up. You must take this into account in the practice of oriental medicine. Our qi is related to the sun and the balance of yin and yang within us.

YIN AND YANG CORRESPONDENCES

The eight trigrams noted above have pairs of opposites.

	Color	Temp	Time	Season*	Dir 1*	Dir 2*	Gender	Movemt	Other
Yang	Bright Red	Warm	Day	Spring Summer	South	East	Left	Male	Up	Dynamic
Yin	Dark Black	Cold	Night	Fall Winter	North	West	Right	Female	Down	Static

* This is representative of *this* hemisphere. If you cross below the equator, this changes.

Some basic concepts that reflect these principles:

- Depression is a Yin disease and stress is worse in yin seasons. (Seasonal Affected Disorder is an example of this.)

- A house's front door in Chinese feng shui (the science of energetic flow through spaces and the effect of that upon life) should face to the south, bringing in energy, fewer germs, wind, cold. If it faces north the energy is drained and the inhabitants face depression.

Where did this south concept come from? From the Yellow Emperor's Classic. When you face south, east is left, west is right.

By the time the system developed the meaning of yin and yang had changed significantly from agricultural terms to represent all that is opposite and complimentary.

CONCEPT OF YIN AND YANG

The concept of Yin and Yang represent two related things or phenomenon which have opposite but complimentary qualities. They can also be represented within *one* thing, as two related aspects of that thing.

As an example, both Yin and Yang can coexist simultaneously within a male (predominantly Yang) body. The same is true for women, who are predominantly Yin – they have definite Yang aspects within that body. Left (Yin) and right (Yang), top (Yang) and bottom (Yin), front (Yin) and back (Yang). All of us have these qualities.

The properties of Yin and Yang are *relative*, not absolute, and can be changed. Three things you need to understand about this

1. Under certain conditions, **Yin and Yang can be changed or switched**.

2. **Yin and Yang can be divided unlimitedly**. Yin and yang are therefore are always dynamic.

3. **Yin and yang contain the *seeds* of each other and one can change into the other** – which is why each half of the tai chi symbol to the right contains the dots of the other's color. Even at the height of yang (represented by the white part of the graphic), the seeds of yin are within. That's what the "I Ching: Book of Changes" is all about.

CONTENT OF YIN AND YANG THEORY

There are four concepts you need to know about Yin and Yang theory:
1. **The opposition of Yin and Yang**
   Left is a copy of right. Top corresponds to bottom. (arms to legs, ie). Opposition is the balance. This is why you use the 4 gates (LI 4 on both left and right hand plus LIV 3 on both left and right foot).

2. **Yin and Yang are interdependent**
   They are opposite, but complementary. Both are needed for wholism and depend upon each other. Without Yin there is no Yang; without Yang there is no Yin. Without light there is no shadow, without shadow you cannot differentiate what "light" is.

3. **Mutual consumption**
   Yin and Yang cycle constantly, a concept represented in the traditional Yin and Yang shape (also called "tai chi symbol"). A continuous cycling of energy is expressed in this symbol. If you're at the top of your career, money, respect…it won't last. But if you're at the bottom, that won't last either! When Yang is more, Yin is less and vice versa.

4. **Inter-transformation**
   Yang is at the top but is changing to Yin. At Summer Solstice, Yang is at its' peak. By the next day, Yin is slowly increasing. These changes are gradual.

   When there is a *severe* or sudden change such as hot one day and very cold the next, there can be repercussions such as illness due to the sudden imbalance of Yin/Yang. This leaves no time to transform naturally. The result is imbalance.

APPLICATION OF YIN-YANG THEORY IN TCM

Yin and yang are *relative* rather than absolute concepts. That means when you compare one thing or aspect to another, one seems more Yang, one seems more Yin in nature. Bear this in mind as you read on.

Yin-Yang Theory relating to the anatomical structure of the human body

I'll summarize with this table and then elaborate afterward.

Area of the body	Yin/Yang correspondence
Top of the body	Yang. Closer to the sun and the heavens
Bottom of the body	Yin. Closer to the earth
Head	The polarity (or highest point) of Yang
Feet	The polarity (or lowest point) of Yin
Left	Yang
Right	Yin
Front	Yin
Back	Yang
Interior of the body	Yin
Exterior of the body	Yang

Head and Foot

There are 361 acupoints on the human body. Of these, there are points that are considered to have a stronger Yin association and some that are considered to have a more Yang association.

Generally speaking, points above the waist are more Yang in nature. The closer a point is to the top of the body, the stronger the Yang is. Du 20, for instance, is considered to be the strongest Yang point and is located at the crown of the head. One of its' other names is "the Sea of Yang." The strongest Yin point on the body is Kidney 1, a point on the sole of the foot just below the ball of the foot.

Left/Right

Left is considered to be more Yang, while right is considered to be more yin. Not only do you have to balance top/bottom, but also left/right.

For those of you with a strong western energetic background, this might be confusing because left is considered more receptive and feminine in this tradition. As my teacher, Dr. Qianzhi Wu said, just remember that women are always right!

Front/Back

The front of the body is more Yin in nature, while the back or dorsal aspect is more Yang in nature. This, too, is springs from China's agricultural traditions. If you were working in the field the part of your body that got the most sun and was thus the most Yang, was your back. The most shaded side is the front, hence the Yin.

Exterior/Interior

The body's exterior is more exposed to sun and is the part that is most active. It is therefore Yang in nature while the interior of the body is considered to be Yin.

Hollow/Solid
Things that are solid are considered to be Yin in nature while things that are hollow ware Yang. The Heart, Liver, Spleen, Lung and Kidney are thought of as "solid" organs and are thus Yin in Chinese medical theory. Hollow organs are the Stomach, Small and Large Intestines, Bladder and Gallbladder and are thus Yang.

> I know this is a bit confusing from the western biomed standpoint, but don't read too much into this right now. There's a LOT more coming!

What are the dividing lines on the body for Yin and Yang? Where does it change from one to the other?

On the trunk
- Hui Yin or meeting of Yin.
  This is the perineum. The Ren 1 acupuncture point is located here, right at the lowest point of the trunk of the body. Anything on the front side of the body from Ren 1 is considered to be more Yin than Yang.

- Hui Yang or meeting of Yang.
  Basically, this is the tip of the tailbone. Bladder 35 is an acupuncture point located here, about 1 cm lateral to the tip of the coccyx. Anything dorsal to this point (on the back) is considered to be more Yang than Yin.

On the extremities

- Tissue closest to the *inside* of the body is yin. The more medial it is, the more yin.

- Tissue closest to the *outside* of the body is Yang. The more lateral it is, the more Yang it is.

You'll see the diagram to the right frequently in Chinese medicine clinics. It's a nice way to illustrate the point locations but is also rooted in the concepts above. The inside of the arm and leg is the medial side and more Yin. The outside or lateral aspect of the extremities are more Yang.

Yin and Yang Theory relating to channel distribution

Yang channels or meridians flow to yang areas while Yin channels flow to Yin areas. There are 15 total channels you will need to learn during this course, 12 of them being the "main" channels. There are 3 Yin channels on the arms, 3 Yin channels on the legs, 3 Yang channels on the arms and 3 Yang channels on the legs. Here is a brief chart detailing the general flow of the channels.

You might want to memorize this. . .

3 hand Yin channels	Go <u>from chest to hand</u> through the medial/palmar aspect of the upper extremeties
3 hand Yang channels	Go <u>from hand to head and face</u> the lateral or dorsal aspect of the upper extremeties.
3 foot Yang channels	Go <u>from face/head to the foot</u> along the lateral or outside aspect of the trunk and lower extremeties.
3 foot Yin channels	Go <u>from foot to abdomen and chest</u> through the medial aspect of the lower extremeties.

The Yang channels of the hand meet the Yang channels of the foot at the head and/or the face. These are converging places of the Yang energy of the body.

Note that the Yin channels of the hand meet the Yin channels of the foot at the chest, a more interior area on the Yin/front aspect of the body.

These are 12 regular channels in the body. Memorize this too…

Hand Taiyin Lung channel	Hand Yangming Large Intestine	Foot Yangming Stomach	Foot Taiyin Spleen
Hand Shaoyin Heart	Hand Taiyang Small Intestine	Foot Taiyang Urinary Bladder	Foot Shaoyin Kidney
Hand Jueyin Pericardium	Hand Shaoyang San Jiao/Triple Burner	Foot Shaoyang Gallbladder	Foot Jueyin Liver

There are anatomical dividing lines separating Yin and Yang on the body, also. When you are standing with your arms at your sides and the palms facing your legs this is how it works:

Thumb	Anterior. Yin in nature
Little finger	Posterior. Yang in nature
Middle finger	Dividing line between Yin and Yang on the upper extremities
Great toe	Anterior. Yin in nature
Little toe	Lateral/posterior. Yang in nature
Middle toe	Dividing line between Yin and Yang channels on the legs.

The line of skin on your palm and the soles of your feet where the skin changes colors and/or textures is a dividing line too. The skin on the palm and on the soles are more Yin in nature than the skin on the back or your hands or on the top of your feet.

Yin-Yang Theory in relation to human physiology

Yin is the material foundation of the human body. Yang is mental and physical activity. The two must be balanced, mind and body, for harmony to exist. By way of example, chewing and digestion are yang things. The body transforms that which you chew and digest into Yin. Yin is then converted into Yang when you perform activities, study, etc.

Rewording this into semi-English: you eat food which would be material or yin, you chew and digest it which expends energy (yang). You store the potential energy, and while it is in its' stored format it is Yin in nature. But then you get up and do something – walk the dog, go study, play Frisbee golf – and you burn the stored resources in order to perform which is again Yang in nature.

YIN-YANG THEORY IN RELATION TO DISEASE PATHOLOGY

Disease is, at the root, a disharmony or imbalance of Yin compared to Yang. We talk about excesses of Yin or Yang as well as deficiencies of Yin and Yang. Excesses and deficiencies have **etiologies** (contributing factors or causes), **mechanisms** (what happens in the body as a result of the etiology), specific **signs and symptoms**, specific **treatment patterns** that work to help relieve the imbalances, and **pattern diagnoses** (clinic speak for each one). You will need to know all of these for both Yin and Yang excesses and deficiencies. Memorize the bejesus out of them!

Excesses

Excesses of Yin and/or Yang are considered to be pathological conditions. An excess means there is *absolutely too much* of either Yin or Yang.

Yang Excess

An excess of Yang in the body is said to be *absolutely too much Yang*. That means it's just too much, too replete, too full. Here's what that looks like.

Etiologies of a Yang excess are the things that can cause this to happen. You'll note that each begins with an introduction into the body of a very heavy Yang influence. When you get to the symptoms and signs portion, note the "big" and heat type signs you see. Even if this is your first exposure to this, you can see some of this.

Etiologies of a Yang excess	
Diet	Spicy and hot foods. Coffee falls into this category as does red ginseng. Both are considered to be very Yang in nature. Both have excellent health benefits, but like all things, in excess or in the presence of other hot and spicy dietary influences, they can cause imbalance.
Invasion of Yang pathogens*	These are external environmental influences. They may come from the natural environment or from manipulation of nature for comfort (air conditioning, heating, etc.). External Yang pathogens are: Wind, Summer Heat, and Fire.
Emotions	Any emotion that is heavily Yang in nature such as anger and irritability can cause an excess of Yang to build in the body. This is why we refer to these people as "hot under the collar!"
Mechanism of a Yang excess	
Mechanism	Yang becomes *absolutely too much*

Signs and Symptoms of a Yang excess	
Face	Red face
Temperature	High fever
Voice	Loud voice
Thirst	Thirst – with a desire to have something cold to drink
Excretions	Dark yellow urination possibly with a hot or burning sensation
	Constipation
	Profuse sweating
Behavior	Manic behavior
Tongue	Red body with yellow, dark yellow, or even brown/black coating
Pulse	Fast – over 90bpm
Treating a Yang Excess	
Sedate	Sedation means removing, eliminating, dispelling, dispersing, cleaning, clearing, and draining. You will see all of these terms in regard to treating excesses in Chinese literature.
	Bloodletting – the fastest and strongest sedation method. There are 10 "spreading" points on the fingertips (you don't use them all at once). Bind the tip of the chosen finger/s, prick it quickly with the proper type of needle and squeeze out 3-5 drops of blood. Bloodletting can also be done at other areas such as Lung 5 (crease of the elbow), Bladder 40 (back of

	the knee on the popliteal crease), and at the apex of the ear.
Pattern diagnosis of a Yang excess	
Clinic speak:	Excessive heat symptoms

*There are six "evils" or external influences that can invade the body: Wind, Cold, Damp, Summer Heat, Fire, and Dryness. Wind, Summer Heat and Fire are considered Yang while the remaining three (cold, damp, and dryness) are considered to be Yin.

Yin Excess

An excess of Yin in the body is said to be *absolutely too much Yin*. That means it's just too much, too replete, too full. Here's what that looks like.

Note the heavy Yin nature of the etiologies as well as all of the excessive cold signs you see in the symptom list.

Etiologies of a Yin excess	
Diet	Dairy, cold foods, slippery foods (like seaweed)
Invasion of Yin pathogens*	These are external environmental influences. They may come from the natural environment or from manipulation of nature for comfort (air conditioning, heating, etc.). External Yin pathogens are: Cold, Dampness, Dryness.
Emotions	Stress and depression
Mechanism of a Yin excess	
Mechanism	Yin becomes *absolutely too much*
Signs and Symptoms of a Yin excess	

Temperature	Chills and an aversion to cold Cold extremities Note: these *cannot be alleviated* by warming therapies! That is a hallmark symptom of a Yin excess.
Tongue	Body is normal, coating could be thin and white
Pulse	Superficial and tight
Treating a Yin Excess	
Sedate	Sedation means removing, eliminating, dispelling, dispersing, cleaning, clearing, and draining. You will see all of these terms in regard to treating excesses in Chinese literature. Always sedate an excess and tonify a deficiency!
	To sedate the excess yin, use moxibustion on the top part of the body is sedation (on the lower part it is tonifying). Use it at the C6 point at the base of the skull on the "Du" points. Also at the L2 vertebra and on the navel. You can also sedate with herbs: make a soup with 3 pieces of onion, 3 pieces of dry chili, and 3 slices of fresh ginger.
Pattern diagnosis of a Yin excess	
Clinic speak:	Excessive cold symptoms

Deficiencies

When there is a deficiency of Yin or Yang there is literally not enough of one or the other. As a result, the other or opposite influence seems to become *relatively too much*, but that's different than excesses where it is *absolutely* too much. This is a 'too much' in that the opposite influence looks like too much, but only when you compare the two.

What?! Let me explain. A deficiency of Yang, for example, would display as what looks like too much Yin. This is kind of like having two 50lb kids on either side of a seesaw. If you take a 50lb kid off of one side and replace that child with a 30lb kid, then the seesaw will sink to the ground on the side where the 50lb kid is. Did that 50lb kid just get too fat? Nope. He or she will just be too heavy when you compare one kid to the other.

When you get to the symptoms for both Yin and Yang deficiencies you'll see that the similar cold and heat signs, but you'll discover that they aren't as excessive as they were in the previous charts. You'll note that there are etiologies, mechanisms, etc to memorize just like you found in the excesses. Again, memorize!!!

Yang Deficiency

Yang deficiency is also referred to as "deficient cold symptoms." Yang (the warm/active/dry part of the body) is too weak so the yin (cold/wet/quiet aspect of the body) becomes relatively too much. Too little warm and relatively too much cold. Kind of like when your shower feels great and then you accidently turn the hot water off.

Etiologies of a Yang Deficiency	
Chronic stage of a cold injured disease	Disease starts at what Zhang Zhongjing described as a Taiyang stage, progresses to a Yangming stage then to a Shaoyang stage. Now it goes to Taiyin → Shaoyin → Jueyin. Taiyang is the strongest in Yang. As the disease progresses, the Yang wanes (kind of burns itself out) and is finally gone all together if the disease is not stopped. A disease is acute if it is less than 3 weeks in the making. Anything

	progressing past that it is considered to be a chronic condition. Chronic conditions are *always deficient conditions*.
Overworking	When you see overworking in relation to yang deficiency the ancient texts are usually referring to too much sexual intercourse and/or masturbation. Isn't that fun to know? Overindulgence of a sexual nature is said to lead to impotence, premature ejaculation, and a low libido.

Mechanism of a Yang Deficiency	
Mechanism	Yin becomes *relatively too much*. If yang is deficient, it fails to control or balance the yin. By comparison, yin becomes *relatively too much*.

Signs and Symptoms of a Yang Deficiency Note: all of these can be relieved with warming therapy! Know this!	
Face	Pale
Temperature	Cold extremities
	Cold pain
	Desire for touching and for warmth
Excretions	Profuse *clear* urination
	Chronic diarrhea around 5am-ish (cock's crow diarrhea)

Sexual s/sx	Impotence
	Premature ejaculation
Energy/behavior	Fatigue
	Poor spirit, very sleepy, might even sleep 10-12 hrs/day
Pulse:	Deep, weak, and slow (less than 60bpm)
Tongue	Pale body, teeth marks (these are scalloped looking edges on the sides where the tongue, which has a case of edema, presses against the teeth).
	Wet or shiny or moist white coating
Treating a Yang deficiency	
Tonify	Always tonify deficiencies and sedate excesses!
	Tonify with warming therapy (or moxa) on lower part of trunk and lower extremities. Typically, this is moxa on Ren 4, 6, 8. Use a piece of fresh ginger, poke holes in it with a needle and place it on Ren 8 (umbilicus). Burn a moxa cone or two on top of it. You could also use sea salt in the umbilicus (make a paper cone out of tissue paper to hold the salt or your patient will be mighty pissed!).
	Warm needle technique. You'll learn more about this in Acupuncture Techniques. Keep card stock or index cards on you for this – cut a slit and place it around

	the base of your needle because you're going to burn a ball of moxa on the top of the needle. The card around the base of the needle will keep the ashes from falling on your patient. (That's lawsuit material, so you definitely need to keep that from happening.)
Pattern diagnosis of a Yang deficiency	
Clinic speak:	Deficient cold symptoms

Yin Deficiency

A depletion of Yin in the body results in the Yang feeling relatively too strong by comparison. Using the shower analogy again, if you are in the shower and the temperature feels perfect then you crank the cold off, you are suddenly scalding hot. You didn't add more hot, you deleted the cold! The result is it feels too hot!

Here we go. More to memorize.

Etiologies of a Yin Deficiency	
Chronic stage of a warm injured disease	Example: summer heat leading to kyphosis (lots o sweatin') leading to dehydration, which is a form of yin deficiency.
Overworking	Especially at night (the Yin time). The human body is really designed to work in the sunshine and sleep at night. Sleep at night builds the yin. Not enough sleep leads to a yin deficiency.
Overindulgence in sexual intercourse	This leads to a loss of Yin due to the loss of fluids during sex. Fluids and blood are Yin in nature – loss of either one can lead to Yin deficiency.

Mechanism of a Yin Deficiency	
Mechanism	Yang becomes *relatively too much.* If Yin is deficient, it fails to control or balance the Yang. By comparison, Yang becomes *relatively* too much.
Signs and Symptoms of a Yin Deficiency	
Deficient heat sx	Night sweats
	Hot flashes
	Palm heat
	Low grade fevers
	"Tidal" fevers – occurring late afternoon around 5-7pm
Facial complexion	Redness only in the cheek or zygomatic areas
Thirst	Not really thirst, but dry mouth/throat. Wants to sip water
Pulse	Deep, thin, fast
Tongue	Thin body, little coating with cracks or "peeled" areas of coating. Coating might even be completely absent – this is called "mirror coat." If there is a coating, it's rough and dry.
Treating a Yang deficiency	
Tonify	Always tonify deficiencies and sedate excesses!
	Tonify and nourish yin with

	acupuncture. Use Kidney 1, Kidney 3, Sp 5, Bl 52, Bl 43
	Dietary and herbal therapies actually work better and are more effective than acupuncture. Bone soup, for instance, which also provides a lot of calcium. Nourish yin, especially during menopause. (You may have noted a lot of menopause like symptoms in the list above.)
Pattern diagnosis of a Yang deficiency	
Clinic speak:	Deficient heat symptoms

All of these patterns and problems relate to Yin and Yang disorders which cause various types of *heat and cold signs and symptoms*. If what you are seeing has no heat or cold specific signs you either didn't clock it right or it's just not Yin or Yang!

Reiterating:
    Excessive Yang = Excessive heat symptoms
    Excessive Yin = Excessive cold symptoms
    Deficient Yang = deficient COLD symptoms
    Deficient Yin = deficient HEAT symptoms

This page intentionally left blank

Chapter 3
Five Element Theory

The Tao begot one.
One begot two.
Two begot three.
And three begot the ten thousand things.

The ten thousand things carry yin and embrace yang.
They achieve harmony by combining these forces.
--Lao Tzu, Tao Te Ching Chapter 42

When the ancient Chinese people looked at their universe they saw the One – the Tao. The Tao gave birth to the two – yin and yang. From yin and yang sprang what Lao Tzu refers to as "the ten thousand things." This is similar to the Judeo-Christian idea. In the beginning God (the One), creates Heaven and Earth (yin and yang) and then the universe is divided again and again (the ten thousand things).

The Five Elements are semi-constants, a further division of the One and of yin and yang, a way to understand the ever-changing nature of the ten thousand things. Like Yin and Yang, where one can transform into the other, the Five Elements cycle, one element feeding from and being born from the previous one and simultaneously giving birth to and feeding the next.

You can study Lao Tzu for decades and still get profound revelations, and I empower you to do so! But first we need to get to how this applies to Chinese medicine. So let's move on.

Five Element Theory Introduction

The big takeaway when thinking about Five Element theory and Chinese medicine is two fold. The focus here is *application* and *interrelationships*. In Chinese, the words used for five element theory are "wu xin."(I won't even attempt that in Chinese characters. I'd just embarrass myself.)

Let's define "wu xin." The term "wu" is the Chinese word for five, which shouldn't be surprising, given we are talking about Five

Element theory. The word "xin" can be translated as element, but can also mean row, street, path. It could even be translated as working or moving. The important thing is to look at the idea of dynamic movement here. This is the idea that it is movement that helps the universe maintain stability by responding and changing as needed to keep the world going like it should.

Five Element theory is used to discuss the five elements and *with* their characteristics and their five element correspondences, their interrelationships, and the movement and flux between them.

THE FIVE ELEMENTS AND THEIR CHARACTERISTICS

The five elements as defined in Chinese philosophies and carrying over into Chinese medicine are Wood, Fire, Earth, Metal, and Water. Let's talk about each one and what their characteristics are.

Wood

Wood, a shapeable element, is attached to the numbers 3 and 8 in Chinese thought. The element of wood includes trees and branches – living wood. The energy of wood expands outward into all directions. The correspondence for wood in the TCM organ system is the organ of the *Liver*. The Liver channel comes up from the feet and branches out into the chest on both sides of the body making a kind of double tree. The energy of the Liver also goes upwards like a tree.

The color correspondence for the element of Wood in TCM is *green*. Think about how trees sprout and grow much faster in the Spring season than in all other seasons. Think too about how you can shape young trees, how you can take harvested wood and both bend and straighten it. Think too about how wind interacts with trees. All of these characteristics apply to the element of Wood and to the Liver, which is the Wood poster child in the human body.

Wood	
Characteristics of Wood	Can be bent
	Can be straightened

Energy and Direction of Wood	Goes upward Expands outward in all directions *except downward*

Fire

Fire, associated with the numbers 2 and 7, gives warmth to the body and is cooks our food, making it more bio-available in most cases. Civilization itself derives from fire.

The energy of fire is warm, hot, and consuming. Flames (and the energy of fire) rises upward. Unsurprisingly, the color of the Fire element is red. Fire corresponds to the Heart organ. The season associated with Fire is summer and it's direction is south.

Fire	
Characteristics of Fire	Warming Flaring upwards
Energy and Direction of Fire	Ascending

Earth

The energy of earth is stable, centering, supportive, and grows everything we need to live. It's cosmological numbers are 5 and 10. How do we acquire and generate energy while we are alive on this earth? The *Neijing* says you can only get energy by breathing air and eating food. In a big city you might feel disconnected from this, but everything we eat and even the air we breathe is given to us from the earth.

You might think of earth as a different color, but in Chinese thought, the color of Earth is yellow.

Earth	
Characteristics of Earth	Permits sowing Permits growing Permits reaping
Energy and Direction of Earth	Neutral and stable

Metal*

Metal, in the Chinese cosmology, has a hard, dense, and heavy energy. It is associated with the cosmological numbers of 4 and 9. Metal, by it's nature, can be molded and hardened. It's color is white and the organ it is associated with is the Lung.

Metal	
Characteristics of Metal	Hard, dense, heavy Can be molded and hardened
Energy and Direction of Metal	Energy is contractile Moves downward and inward

*Metal? I thought that was weird at first. I studied tarot and some other esotericky type stuff before I studied Chinese medicine. The whole metal as an element thing threw me off for a while. Then I realized that the element of air is often represented as a sword in western esoteric thought. That helped me remember this element. Maybe it'll help you too.

Water

The number one element is water, according to the esteemed Dr. Qianzhi Wu. When you are conceived, it is in the fluid element that characterizes what's happening for you in those first months of life. This sets the tone for your whole physical existence. Our bodies are composed of 70-75% water and it corresponds to conception, gestation, and the body. The numbers 1 and 6 in the Chinese cosmology are associated with water.

Water is moistening (I know, duh) and flows downward (also duh). Water is heavy in nature and is characterized by the color black. Black? Yes. Think about a very deep ocean. The deeper it is, the blacker the color. The organ that corresponds to this element is Kidney.

Water	
Characteristics of Water	Moistening Heavy
Energy and Direction of Water	Descending downward

Memorize the following charts. You're going to need them often, not just for this class, but for the rest of your Foundations education, Diagnostics studies, and in clinical practice. Trust me on this one.

Five Elements in Nature						
	Season	Climate	Direction	Color	Taste	Smell
Wood	Spring	Wind	East	Green	Sour	Rancid
Fire	Summer	Heat	South	Red	Bitter	Burned
Earth	Late Summer	Damp	Middle	Yellow	Sweet	Sweetish
Metal	Autumn	Dryness	West	White	Pungent	Rank
Water	Winter	Cold	North	Black	Salty	Putrid

Five Elements in The Human Body						
	Zang/Yin	Fu/Yang	Sense Organ	Body Tissue	Emotions	Sounds
Wood	Liver	Gallbladder	Eye	Sinews	Angry	Shouting
Fire	Heart	Small Intestine	Tongue	Vessels	Joy	Laughter
Earth	Spleen	Stomach	Mouth	Muscle	Worry	Singing
Metal	Lung	Large Intestine	Nose	Skin	Grief	Crying
Water	Kidney	Bladder	Ear	Bone	Fear	Groaning

Notes about these charts
1. In a perfect world this would be one chart joined by the Wood, Fire, Earth, Metal, and Water in the middle, but Kindle Textbook Creator just couldn't figure out how to make this page flip sideways. Sorry, folks.

2. Wood: since Liver opens to the eyes an is associated wit this sensory organ, crying and tears are cleansing to the Liver organ and to the channel.

3. Fire has on overcooked smell and taste, like charred food.

4. Earth is associated with sweetness, like grains. I don't readily associate grain with sweet, but if you cook rice or even popcorn and taste it without any flavorings you can detect a very light sweetness to the grains. Grain is also the substance from which a lot of fermented drinks are made, letting you know that there is enough sugar in grain to ferment!

5. Water and the Kidney/Bladder are associated with the lower openings: urethra and anus. Kidneys control water in the body. Water is associated with the color black because when water is very deep it is black. As for the putrid smell, think about any fish market or even the fish areas at grocery stores like Central Market. Kidney opens to the ears – long ear lobes are a sign of good Kidney essence and therefore a long life. Conversely, degradation of the Kidney can result in tinnitus/ear ringing and decline in the ability to hear.

6. Late summer is also called Long Summer. It is the end of summer, beginning of autumn. Humidity is higher, more clouds, more rain, which sounds a lot like August/September in Texas. Ugh. Nasty. Don't miss it one bit.

Really. Seriously. **Memorize these charts**. Be able to write it out. Make blanks for yourself –fill them out over and over again until you can do it in your sleep. One student had it laminated at an office store and used it like a write board to practice. Again, just sayin.'

INTERRELATIONSHIPS BETWEEN THE FIVE ELEMENTS

It's not enough to know the individual elements. That's great, but what is equally important in medicine is how they interact together.

Generating Sequence

This means that each element generates another and also originates from the elements before it. You will see slight differences in the charts you find online. Some start with fire at the top, some with earth. The one I got from my professors always had Wood/Liver at the top of the chart, so that's what this one looks like too.

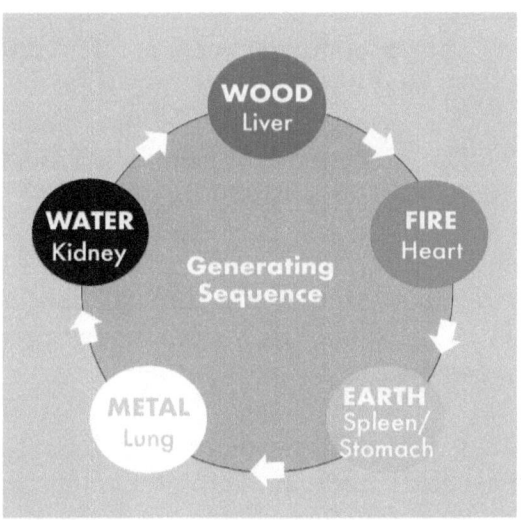

Look at the arrows pointing from one element to the next. This is the ***natural and healthy order of the flow of energy*** from one to the next.

Let's start with Fire, even though that element is not at the top. Fire burns and generates ashes, which feed the element of Earth. Earth and fire in turn generate metal. Metal/air generates Water, which then feeds the element of Wood. Wood then becomes fuel for the Fire.

Wait a minute. How does Metal give birth to water? Here's how the association was explained to me:

- When Metal is heated to the appropriate temperature (iron ore melts at 2750°F/1510°C), it converts from a solid to a fluid.

- Metal is found underground and very often near a creek or river and generally has a close groundwater source. Mining is often plagued by problems of water filling up the mining shafts.

- Water condenses on metal when the weather changes.

> The generating element is referred to as the **Mother** element.
>
> The element that *is generated* from the Mother is called the **Son** or **Child**.

Remember this "Mother and Son" relationship. Energy by its' very nature should flow from mother (generator) to son (or generated).

A principle you will hear more about later: for deficiencies of a given element/organ, tonify the mother element.

Controlling or Checking Sequence

In the controlling sequence, one elements controls another element and is likewise, controlled by another element. Here's another version of the diagram above showing the Controlling Sequence.

Do you see the star shape formed by the black arrows in the center of the elements? This is the **natural and healthy order** of the flow of controlling energy through the elements. In this manner, each elements checks or controls another element so that energy doesn't overgrow.

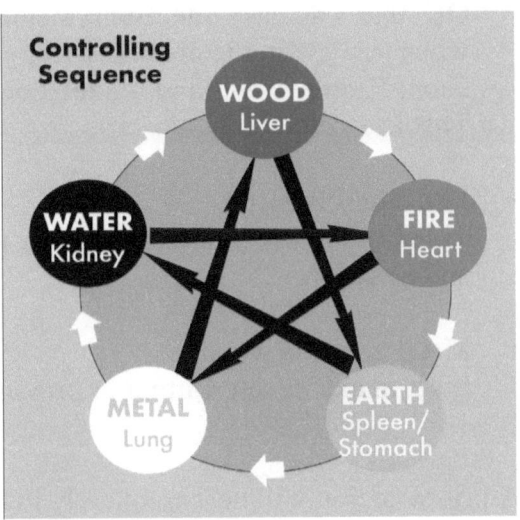

Both the Generating and the Controlling sequenences are *normal and healthy*. The control sequence is one element keeping another in check or in balance. You'll see this concept again when you study Four Needle Technique in your acupuncture studies. In that context, it is referred to as the Ko element or channel.

Here's how each element controls another.

- Wood controls earth.
  Think about tree roots gripping into earth. Areas that have a lot of trees generally have less soil erosion for this reason. But by the same token, we've probably all seen a tree, however small, growing up from a rock. Trees and their roots can also break down rock/earth.

- Earth controls water
  Think about dams holding back water, about water

being contained between river banks, and even how the structure of earth below a body of water can modify how water moves. This is true for lakes and rivers, but also for oceans and seas.

- Water controls fire.
  OK, that's an easy one. But remember this imagery when you get to the classes where you start talking about Kidney/water and it's relationship to Heart/fire. This is a crucial relationship.

- Fire controls metal.
  Think of the fire in a forge making metal malleable and workable.

- Metal controls wood.
  Like an axe or saw cutting or pruning a tree.

A principle you will hear frequently in Five Element approaches to treatment: for an excess of a given element/organ, sedate the Son or Child element.

> Both the Generating and Controlling sequences are normal and natural sequences and are mutually needed to maintain balance.

Over-controlling or Over-checking

While the control sequence is normal, it can *over*-control (which you might also see as "over-check") when the balance is broken. Over-controlling or over-checking is a ***pathological*** process of the controlling sequence. The over-control follows the same sequence as the controlling cycle, so Wood could over-check Earth, Earth could over-check Water, etc.

When an element over-checks another, the one which is over-controlled becomes weak. For example, if the Wood element is too strong/too much, it will over-control the Earth element, rendering it weak. In the clinic you will see this as an excess of the Wood element or the Liver (often referred to as Liver Qi Stagnation) beating up on the Spleen and Stomach (the Earth Element) and causing digestive issues.

(The whole concept reminds me of a micro-managing super controlling boss I once had who *did* give me acid indigestion, now that I think about it!)

Counterchecking

This too is a *pathological* process of the controlling sequence. The counterchecking sequence also refers to the control relationship between elements, but the flow of energy is reversed. For example, instead of wood affecting earth, it would *insult* the metal element which normally controls it. This is a backflow of energy, shown by the red arrows in the diagram. No es bueno.

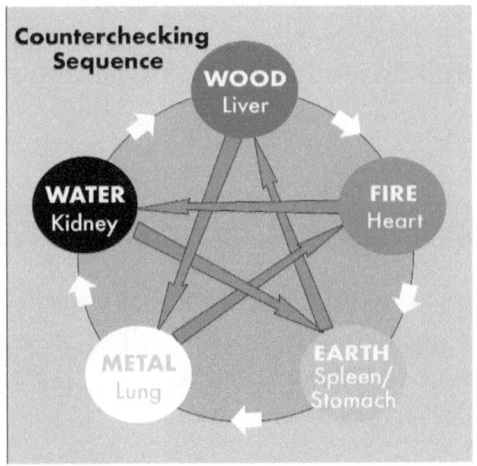

Insulting

This *pathological* process of the generating sequence. It refers to a child or son element insulting the parent/mother. As an example, the mother element of fire is supposed to generate earth, but in this case the earth element insults fire. This is like a kid rebelling against his/her parent. You can see the pathological flow of energy in the red arrows going counterclockwise below.

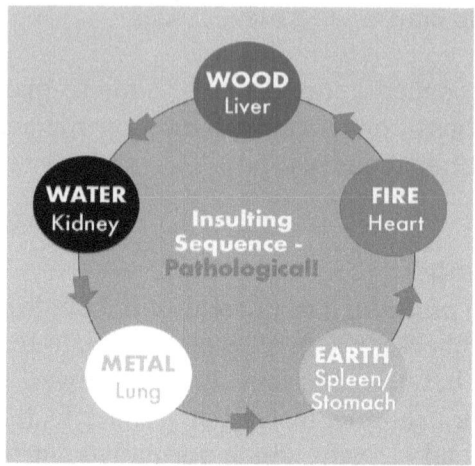

Overacting

This pathological process of the generating sequence refers to a mother element overacting on the child/son. This is like an over controlling mother who is so extreme she raises a dysfunctional child.

APPLICATION OF FIVE ELEMENT THEORY IN TCM

Now that you've got some of the theory under your belt, let's talk about how it applies in Chinese Medicine. All of these points together point to the TCM concept of wholism – that all things are interrelated and cannot really be separated.

Five Element Theory in Physiology

In terms of physiology, Five Element Theory helps you understand internal organ functions.

TCM does not advocate the dissection of bodies like western medicine does. It's considered very disrespectful to the body. In Daoism, from whence oriental medical theory sprang, there are two souls (three, depending on what source you read): the Hun or yang aspect that returns to heaven or the great cosmos upon death and the Po which is the yin aspect of the soul. The Po is a product of earth and returns to the earth upon death. You don't disrespect the earth element of a body with purposeful dissection when a human being dies. That just ain't cool.

Instead, you pay attention to, observe, and research the outside body. It's sort of the Sherlock Holmes type of medicine where every visible, smell-able, hear-able, and touch-able detail is important. By adding up the clues you see in the pulse, the tongue, the demeanor of the person, what you find when you palpate the body and question the client, etc., you get a very good picture of what is happening inside.

Five Element Theory connects the 5 Yin organs to the whole body together

TCM pays the most attention to Yin (also referred to as Zang) organs. The Yin organs have a paired organ, the Yang or Fu organ. Though the primary emphasis is placed on the Yin organs, the relationship between Yin/Zang and Yang/Fu organs is extremely important. They are even referred to as wife/husband pairs in some literature. .

For example, if you have a Gallbladder related problem, you would treat the Liver channel also because Liver (yin) and Gallbladder (yang) correspond and are interrelated. (A note about the Liver: eyes are connected to the Liver – look back at your chart! – and Liver controls the flow of emotions, so when you get sad, you cry which cleanses the Liver.)

Five Element Theory connects the internal environment with the external environment

The internal environment is the *organ* side of the Five Element chart and includes not just the organs, but the whole body. The external environment is the *nature* side of the chart. The external environment deeply affects the internal environment of the body. Diseases are seasonal for this reason. We like to think we exist in a little climate-controlled bubble, unaffected by the outside world, but we don't. My grandfather could tell you when a storm was coming before the weatherman could because his knees would ache and an old scar would itch. He was rarely wrong.

When you plant a garden you may develop it, plant it, even put a wall up around it, but the environment external to that garden will still greatly affect it nonetheless. If there's a drought or a freeze or too much rain it's going to affect that garden unless you take measures to protect it. The body is the same!

Five Element Theory explains the internal organ relationship

Chinese medicine doesn't focus on individual function of the organs, but on their inner/inter- relationships. And please remember the organ consists of more than just the tissues that make up that physical organ – the "organ" wasn't even originally named for an organ, but for a whole range of functions. Spleen is my favorite. In the old literature it isn't called "Spleen" (some French guy mistranslated it actually, and the mistranslation stuck), but was referred to as the Sea of Grain. Later on this will make SO much more sense to you!

We touched on this a little bit earlier in this chapter. The organs and elements are intimately connected through the generating and control sequence, one creating another, being created by another, controlling and being controlled by another.

Five Element Theory in Pathology

We touched on this a bit too. Look back at the sequences and you'll see that only two are healthy and normal – the Generating and Controlling sequences. You might remember too that the pathological energetic relationships can be based in the Generating sequence and in the Controlling sequence. Pathological versions of these sequences create sickness and dis-ease.

Let's take a look at the pathologies – the things that go wrong.

Pathological transmission according to Generating Sequence

- Mother affecting son.
  This is the overbearing parent suppressing the child element which then becomes weak. This follows the generating sequence in energy flow, so Fire (as a mother element) would affect Earth (it's corresponding son element), Earth would affect Metal, etc.

- Son affecting Mother
  In this case, the child element rebels and affects the mother element. Taking Fire and Earth as an example, this would be Earth affecting or rebelling against the Mother.

  If you can understand and uncover a patient's medical history, you can understand which of their problems came first and it can give you a clue as to whether Mother is affecting Son or Son is affecting Mother. Why is this important? Because mother affecting son is the normal flow of energy through the cycle. If the cycle has somehow been reversed and the son is affecting the mother, the prognosis for the patient is not as good.

Pathological transmission according to the Controlling Sequence

This is the five pointed star transmission of energy – Earth to Water, Water to Fire, Fire to Metal, Metal to Wood, Wood to Earth.

- Overcontrolling
  The control element is overbearing and over-controls it's correspondent element. So if metal over-controls wood, wood then becomes weak. This still follows the natural flow of energy between the control/controlled elements, but is an out-of-balance

condition resulting in disease/disharmony.

- Insulting
  This also causes disease/disharmony, but the energy flow is in reverse. Instead of Metal controlling Wood, Wood now insults Metal.

Let's overlay the corresponding organs over this: metal corresponds to lung. Wood corresponds to Liver. If Liver/wood is too strong it insults Lung/metal. Cirrhosis of the Liver, for example, eventually results in coughing out blood from the Lungs due to portal hypertension.

In this diagram, the organ, Liver/Wood is too strong and throws it's energy outward at another organ or organs.

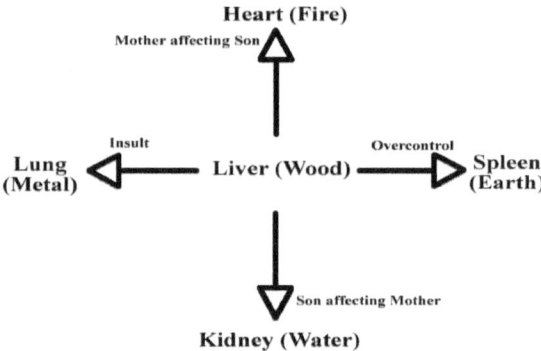

All or some of the scenarios above can occur. Here's what might happen with each.

- If Liver/wood over-controls Spleen/earth digestive problems result.

- If Liver/wood as the son affects the mother of Kidney/water, the result can be ascites – water in the abdomen – or edema in the feet or ankles.

- If Liver/wood insults the Lung/metal, it can result in epistaxis (nose bleed) or portal hypertension.

- Liver/wood as the son affecting the mother of Heart/fire can express as mental symptoms such as delirium or hallucinations, or as blood disorders.

You might want to do this exercise for all Yin organs to help you understand what could go wrong in these scenarios.

In this diagram, the organ has become too weak, so the energies of the surrounding organs overwhelm the weak organ…it's nothing personal, just the way energy flows. In A & P you will encounter this concept as the concentration gradient.

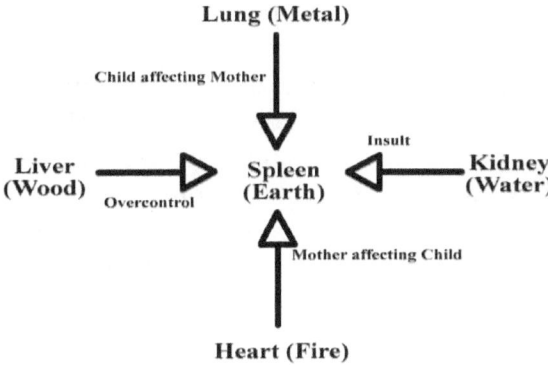

FIVE ELEMENT THEORY FOR DIAGNOSIS AND TREATMENT

In terms of diagnosis, a thorough patient history can help you understand what came first in the patient's health and then what is affecting, insulting, over-controlling, etc. In terms of treatment, Five Element theory can help you craft great ways to treat dysfunction. Generating sequences gone awry, for instance, can lead to deficiencies and excesses. When you see Controlling sequences gone badly you know right away that you can sedate excesses and tonify deficiencies.

Treatment principles according to dysfunctional generation sequences

Generating sequence dysfunction lead to deficiencies and excesses. You will see the principles below in the four needle technique which you will encounter in Point Location and Energetics materials.

- Deficiency
  To treat a deficiency, the principle is to **tonify the mother element.**

  Example: a patient with digestive problems, indicating Spleen problems, may also have a soft voice and a chronic cough, indicating Lung dysfunction. Since the Spleen is the mother element and the Lung is the son element, this indicates that the Spleen problem is causing a weakness in the Lung. The principle of tonify the mother for deficiencies applies here, so you tonify Spleen to fix both the digestive and the Lung dysfunctions.

- Excess
  To treat an excess, the principle is to sedate the Son/Child element. This gives more energy to the Mother element in the sequence.

Treatment principles according to dysfunctional Controlling Sequence

Simultaneously sedate the excesses while tonifying the deficiencies.
Xiao Yao San has 4 ingredients to sedate the Liver while tonifying the Spleen.

A COUPLE OF CASE STUDIES

Case Discussion 1
A person suffers from digestive disorders with symptoms of epigastric pain, decreased appetite, gas, bloating, nausea, vomiting,

alternating constipation and diarrhea. These symptoms are caused by so called Liver Qi Stagnation: depression, anger, stress, and frustration.

Question: According to the Five Element Theory, what is the transmission of the disease?

> Answer: Liver was affected first, which then began to affect spleen. This would be Liver Over-controlling Spleen. Note: if there is pain or discomfort above the umbilicus/belly button = Stomach. If there is pain *below* the umbilicus = Spleen.

Case Discussion 2
A middle-aged male patient suffers from palpitations, dream disturbed sleep, pale face, fatigue, poor memory and bad concentration. These symptoms have lasted for a period of six months and are considered to be a heart blood deficiency. He also had a poor appetite, chronic diarrhea with occasional nausea for over 2 years. An OM practitioner diagnosed this as a spleen qi deficiency. The patient felt that his blood deficiency was a result of the digestive disorder.

Question: What is the connection between these two problems?

> Answer: The patient has had a spleen qi deficiency for 2 years – problems in the 3arth element. Now in the last 6 months he has had problems in the heart/fire zone. This is son affecting mother.

Case Discussion 3
A 35 year old male patient has been suffering from excessive heart fire for over 10 days with tongue ulcers, burning pain in the tongue, thirst, irritability and insomnia. Two days ago, the patient started to have anger, short temper, red eyes, which is a condition called Liver Fire Flaring Up. In addition to this, the patient coughed badly with a little blood in the mucus.

Question: How do you explain the transmission of the symptoms according to the Five Element Theory?

>Answer: Son (heart) affecting mother (liver). Also, the patient is coughing blood, a Lung problem. Could also be heart/fire overacting upon lung/metal.

Sidebar:
A comprehensive diagnosis in Chinese medicine consists of:
1. The OM diagnosis
2. The Western/Biomed diagnosis
3. Differential/pattern diagnosis
4. Properties – is it a single excess or deficiency or a combination of excess and deficiency? If so, what percentage of each?
5. Principles of treatment (i.e., sedate the excess, clear Heart fire, etc…)
6. Methods of treatment: acu points, herbal formulas, cupping, guasha, etc.

Chapter 4
Zangfu Theory

We touched on this briefly in Chapter 3 in the Five Element discussion. Zang refers to Yin organs in the body and Fu refers to Yang organs. You cannot speak of the vital functions of the body without knowing Zangfu theory well.

There are two meanings to Zangfu. One meaning is "internal organ" and the other is "hide." Both apply as the internal organs are hidden within.

Zang Xiang is another term in TCM that means Zangfu. This term means both "image" and "sign and symptoms showing from superficial areas."

The methodology in TCM is to get to know internal organ functions by looking at signs and symptoms on the superficial body. Without opening and examining the body, external signs will reveal with is internal. The exterior *image* reveals the condition of the *internal organs*. And the image, the presentation, is the most important thing in Chinese medicine.

> The purpose of Zangfu theory is to discuss internal organ functions (physiological functions), pathological changes, and the interrelationships of the 12 internal organs through the signs and symptoms (image) showing from the superficial areas.

Note: Some of the way this is presented will very likely be contrary to what you will read in the Maciocia books. My Chinese professors both loved and loathed him simultaneously. Also, I should tell you that Zangfu was heavily emphasized in the school I attended, which was predominantly an herbal school, so Zangfu is a huge deal there. In other schools you might see more emphasis on Five Element theory or other theories.

THE ZANGFU CATEGORIES

There are 3 types of internal organs and meridians/channels: yin (or zang), yang (or fu) and extraordinary organs. In most Chinese medicine schools you will see the most attention focused on the regular organs and meridians. Bear in mind that the *Yellow Emperor's Internal Classic* names five yin and six yang organs for a total of eleven, leaving the Pericardium out entirely. It was added later.

Zang/Yin Organs

The Zang organs, or the yin organs, are considered to be "solid organs." They get the primary emphasis in Zangfu theory. They are:

Organ name	Channel name
Lung	Hand Taiyin
Spleen	Foot Taiyin
Heart	Hand Shaoyin
Kidney	Foot Shaoyin
Pericardium	Hand Jueyin
Liver	Foot Jueyin

Fu/Yang Organs

The Fu, or yang organs, are considered to be hollow organs in that they contain things – for a while – then empty out and repeat. That will make sense to you based on the western anatomy you know. . . until you get to the San Jiao which I will explain in a bit. They are:

Organ name	Channel name
Large Intestine	Foot Yangming
Stomach	Foot Yangming
Small Intestine	Hand Taiyang
Urinary Bladder	Foot Taiyang
San Jiao*	Hand Shaoyang
Gallbladder	Foot Shaoyang

*What the heck is a San Jiao?! There's no western equivalent really. The San Jiao, also called the Triple Burner or Triple Warmer, is like a water pumping system in that it is the controller of the movement of water throughout the body. If you think of it using this plumbing metaphor, you can see that it is truly a hollow organ.

San means three and Jiao refers to the three major divisions of the body. These three sections are the Upper Jiao, Middle Jiao, and Lower Jiao They are used not only to talk about how water flows in the body, but also as a general reference to anatomical location in Chinese literature.

- Upper Jiao
  Refers to the breathing diaphragm and all tissues above it – head, chest, lungs, heart, and five sense organs.

- Middle Jiao
  The area from the umbilicus to the breathing diaphragm. This includes the Spleen, Stomach, Liver and Gallbladder... most of the time. Sometimes you'll see the Liver/Gallbladder pair bundled into the lower jiao. Try not to think about that too much right this second!

- Lower Jiao
  Everything below the umbilicus. Small intestine, Large intestine, Bladder, Kidneys. (OK, and occasionally the Liver and Gallbladder pair.

The Extraordinary Organs – Heng Zhi Fu.

Sometimes these are called the Strange Organs. They aren't really that strange, they just aren't connected with the 12 major meridians. These special cases, however are intimately connected with the Eight Extraordinary *Vessels* (Du, Ren, Chong, Dai, Yin/Yang Wei, Yin/Yang Qiao), all of which originate from the uterus in women or from the semen palace (testes) in men. The six Extraordinary Organs are:

- Brain
- Uterus
- Marrow
- Bone

- Vessels
- Gallbladder*

* An explanation as to why Gallbladder is classified in both the Fu organs and the Extraordinary Organs is coming. Hang in there.

THE FUNCTIONS OF THE INTERNAL ORGANS

Do yourself a favor - memorize the functions of the internal organs – Zang, Fu, and Extraordinary! This discussion is on the general rather than the specific functions of the organs. We'll get to the specifics later. As you read, note that the general energy of the Yin organs is upward moving while the general energy of the Yang organs is downward moving.

The common functions for Zang/Yin or solid organs and for the Fu/Yang or hollow organs is as follows.

Yin organs *generate* and *produce* vital substances

These vital substances are Blood, Qi, Essence, and Body Fluids.

Vital Substance	Where it comes from
Blood	Generated by the Spleen and Heart with the help of the Lungs and Kidneys
Qi	Generated by Lungs, Spleen, and Kidneys
Body Fluids	Produced by the Spleen, Stomach, Small Intestine, and Large Intestine
Essence	Produced from the Kidneys and Spleen

Yin organs *store* vital substances

Yin Organs are static in that they are solid and store vital substances.

Liver	Stores Blood
Kidneys	Store Essence
Qi	Stored in all Yin/Zang organs
Body Fluids	Stored in all Yin/Zang organs

> Side note: While the Maciocia book says that Shen is also a vital substance, Dr. Wu disagrees and says that Shen is Yang in nature. Maciocia probably places this here because Shen is one of the 3 treasures.

Fu/Yang organs receive and hold water and food
The digestive organs are all connected together: Stomach, Small Intestine, Large Intestine, Gallbladder. The Urinary Bladder is connected to the digestive tract via the San Jiao, a Yang organ paired with the Pericardium.

When the Stomach is full, the Small and Large Intestines should be *empty*. Conversely, when the Small and Large Intestines are full the Stomach should be empty.

Fu/Yang organs transport water and food

These organs are more dynamic than Zang/Yin organs. Food and water should not stop at any organ. If any of these organs stop their *downward* moving energy and store the substances that are supposed to be passing through, them inflammation results.

Have you ever eaten a big meal that just wouldn't digest or gotten a stomach bug? Both of those things can result in the *upward* or dysfunctional movement of Stomach energy and the result is vomiting. Yeah. Down is good in that case!

Each channel associated with an organ has a point called a He Sea point. These points are located around the knees and elbows. The yang channels of the upper body, Large Intestine, San Jiao, and Small Intestine have He Sea points around the elbows, but they also have Lower He Sea points on the lower extremities. Actually, all Yang channels have He Sea and Lower He Sea points. This is due to the importance of the downward moving nature of these organs/channels.

Function of the Extraordinary Organs

The only function of the Extraordinary Organs is to store vital substances. Together with the eight Extraordinary *Vessels* they work as reservoirs and are located deeply in the body to store Qi, Blood, Essence, and Fluids. Look at the chart below to see the alternative names and how that reflects this storage reservoir idea.

Brain	Sea of Marrow
Uterus	Blood chamber*
Liver	Blood chamber*
Sea of Blood	Blood chamber*

*Yes, there are three. Lots of blood going on here.

These are "Extraordinary Organs" because they do not fit into either Yin or Yang categories and do not produce substances, yet are hollow (like the Yang organs and *do* store substances (like the Yin organs). They have yin organ functions, but yang organ shape.

Ok, this is a good spot to give you that explanation I promised about why the Gallbladder both a Yang and and Extraordinary organ.

- It's Yang because it *does* involve digestion and the overall downward movement.

If the Gallbladder is full of stones or sludge it will

negatively affect digestion. Why? Because it releases bile, which breaks down fats.

- It's a bit Yin because the Gallbladder stores and holds (bile in this case), but cannot produce.

Bile in Chinese medicine (chapter 6 of the *Neijing*) is considered to be one of the vital substances, "zhongjing" or central essence. In biomedicine you see that bile is produced by the liver then is moved to the gallbladder for concentration and excretion.

Another note on the Gallbladder in Chinese medicine theory: it decides part of your personality – to have a "big gallbladder" is a Chinese idiom usage is to say that someone is very brave. Someone with a 'small gallbladder' is very timid, easily startled or frightened.

This page intentionally left blank

CHAPTER 5
Heart and Small Intestine

This chapter begins an expansion of and detailed look into more specifics of Zangfu theory. We're starting with the Heart (Zang/Yin) and Small Intestine (the coupled Fu/Yang organ). The Heart *governs* Blood and is dependent upon Qi to fuel the energy of the Heart and the movement of the Blood through the body. (Remember that the Liver *stores* Blood.)

GENERAL INTRODUCTION TO THE HEART

The Heart is the most important organ

The Heart is referred to as the Ruler, Emperor and Monarch of all internal organs. And this is true! You cannot live without the Heart. In Chinese culture, rank is very important. To say that the Heart is the Monarch is to give it the highest status. For this reason some schools of Chinese medicine say that one must not needle points on the Heart channel as this will deplete the Heart energy. These schools recommend needling the Pericardium channel instead.

Location of the Heart

The Heart is located in the Upper Jiao on the left side of the chest above the diaphragm. It looks like a reverse lotus, the holy flower in Buddhism. The Pericardium is a membrane covering the surface of the Heart. Chinese medicine regards the Pericardium as a yin organ separate from but closely tied to the heart – like a Prime Minister. Needling on the Pericardium channel will transfer the benefits directly to the Heart. For this reason, Pericardium 6, 7 and 8 are used often for heart problems.

Physiological Functions of the Heart

All functions of the Heart are based upon Heart qi, the pushing energy of the Heart.

There are ten physiological functions to know regarding the Heart. Know the functions well. Here they are in summary with deeper discussion and explanation to follow. *Memorize these 10 functions!*

1. The Heart governs Blood
2. The Heart controls the blood vessels
3. The Heart manifests in the facial complexion
4. The Heart houses the Shen
5. The Heart is related to joy
6. The Heart opens to the tongue
7. The Heart controls sweating
8. The Heart controls dreaming
9. The Heart loathes heat
10. The Heart controls speech

The Heart Governs the Blood

The Heart governs the Blood in two ways.

Heart qi *transforms* blood
That is to say, the Heart Qi transforms *stuff* into Blood. Food and drink go from the Stomach, which ripens and rots what is ingested, then passes the goodies to the Small Intestine which has the function of separating out the good from the not so good. The not-so-good is also called "turbid" in Chinese medicine speak. Once the good stuff is extracted, that energy then goes to the Spleen. The Spleen absorbs the essence from the food and sends this *ying* or *nutritive qi* up to the Heart. This ying qi is converted by the Heart into "red body fluids," which is how the classic texts refer to Blood.

A dysfunctional Spleen or Heart may not have enough energy produce the building blocks that are then used to generate Blood. Ergo, if you want to nourish Blood, you also have to tonify the Qi, especially the Heart qi.

Heart Qi, the pushing energy of the Heart, *transports* the Blood
This is related to both Heart Qi and Heart yang. Yang and Qi are actually closely associated with Qi and is the active principle of energy. Heart Yang/Qi pushes the Heart, and therefore the Blood, circulating it throughout the body to nourish the internal organs, extremities and the five sensory organs.

If the Heart qi is dysfunctional or deficient, it can manifest as a pale face or pallor, pale tongue, fatigue, and cold extremities. Secondary symptoms can include purple face and lips indicating a stagnation in the flow of blood, and chest pain with stuffiness in the chest.

The Heart controls the blood vessels

This is true in the Western medical model as well. The state of the Heart energy is reflected in the state of the blood vessels. The vessels depend upon the Heart's Qi and Blood to both nourish the vessels and fill them. Because the Heart Qi pushes the circulation, if the Qi is strong, the vessels will be too. If the Heart Qi is weak, the pulse is weak and irregular.

Good blood circulation requires open blood vessels with no obstructions, sufficient blood volume and quality in the vessels to move (which is why deficient blood shows as a thin, weak pulse) and a strong enough Heart Qi to generate a normal blood flow.

The Heart manifests in the complexion

Though it distributes Blood all over the body, it is in the facial complexion that the Heart truly manifests. A normal complexion, reflecting good Heart function is rosy and lustrous. Poor heart function shows as pale, dull white or bright white.

Heart Dysfunction	Correspondent facial complexion
Deficient Blood or Deficient Heart Qi	Pale or bright white
Blood stagnation	Purplish or bluish
Heart heat	Red

The Heart houses the Shen (the Mind)

Mind is called *shen* in Chinese medicine and culture. Shen is also sometimes translated as the *spirit* of a body. There are 2 meanings for *shen*:

- Narrow meaning - mental activities, including emotions, consciousness, memory, thinking, and sleep.

- Broad meaning – the comprehensive expression of a live human body, including facial complexion, eye movement, conversation, answers to questions, speech, mannerisms, etc. All of this reflects the energy and different expressions of a body: inactive and withdrawn or hyperactive with lots of talking.

While Blood is Yin in nature, Shen is Yang in nature. The *Heart needs adequate blood in order to nourish/hold the shen*. Physiologically, if the Heart has enough Qi and Blood, a person can think, concentrate and remember well, and sleep soundly. To increase memory, especially short term memory, and concentration focus on tonifying Heart Blood, since a strong Heart is the hoe to a strong mind.

Because Shen is also closely linked with emotions, strong Heart Qi and Blood will also yield a happier person. Poor Heart function leads to poor spirit, sadness and depression, especially when the Heart Qi and Blood are blocked.

Pathological expressions of poor or deficient Heart qi are poor memory, bad concentration, poor sleeping, pale face. Pathological expressions of excess conditions of the Heart or Blood are Shen disturbances such as mania. Most often Heart fire will cause manic behavior while Heart Blood deficiency will cause insomnia with dream-disturbed sleep.

If you wish to nourish the Shen, tonify the Heart and the Heart Blood.

Each of the Five Yin/Zang organs is "in charge" of a certain mental activity or aspect of the emotional self.

Organ	Emotion
Heart	Mind or Shen
Liver	Ethereal soul (Hun)
Lungs	Corporeal soul (Po)
Kidney	Will power (Zhi)
Spleen	Thought (Yi)

The Heart is related to and controls joy

Joy in balance makes the mind peaceful and relaxed, benefiting the nutritive (ying) and defensive (wei) qi, encouraging these 2 forms of qi to relax and flow well. Joy in excess however can injure the heart: this would be mania or schizophrenia. All emotions are considered physiologically normal until out of balance. When out of balance they become pathological and cause disease.

The Heart opens to the Tongue

The tongue is an offshoot of the Heart. The color, form and appearance of it are all controlled by the Heart. Here are some examples:

Heart Dysfunction	Correspondent tongue expression
Heat in the Heart	Tip of the tongue is very red
Heart Blood deficiency	Tongue body is very pale
Blood stagnation	Tongue body is very stiff

Organ conditions other than those of the Heart are also reflected in the status of the tongue. The Spleen channel, for example, goes to the root or undersurface of the tongue. The sides of the tongue show problems in the Liver and Gallbladder. The back of the top surface of the tongue can show problems in the Lower Jiao, etc.

Heart qi also communicates through the tongue. There are 5 tastes: sweet, salty, sour, pungent, and bitter (some also throw in bland here). If you can taste all 5, your heart *and* spleen are functioning well. Because the Heart governs blood and houses Shen this is reflected in the movement of the tongue. If a person stutters, the problems are of the Heart *and* Kidney. Stiffness of the tongue can occur after a stroke causing aphasia. Flaccidity of the tongue can reflect Heart deficiency.

The Heart controls sweating

Other organs do too, especially the Lung, but in different ways. The Heart's role in controlling sweating has to do with its function of governing Blood. Blood is a combination of Body Fluid and *ying* or nutritive qi. Sweat, as a part of the Body Fluids, comes from the spaces between the skin and muscles.

The Heart can affect sweat by controlling Blood and Body Fluids. If the Heart Qi or Yang is insufficient, a person may sweat profusely. By way of example, patients with congestive heart failure often have profuse sweating as a symptom. Western medicine acknowledges that to loose too much fluid through dehydration or profuse sweating will affect the heart and blood.

Very important: if there is a Heart Blood deficiency, *do not* promote sweating! These deficiencies will render the heart incapable of holding the fluids together with the blood and it will leak out in the form of sweat.

The Heart controls dreaming

All dreams relate to the Heart and are a manifestation of Shen and reflect the status of the Shen. If your Heart is balanced, you will sleep well. If not, you may experience insomnia, superficial sleep, and/or dream disturbed sleep. Vivid dreams and dream disturbed sleep are abnormal phenomenon rather than basic garden variety dreaming in which you likely won't remember the dreams even if you remember dreaming. When dreams disturb your sleep, they will wake you up, scare you, or be anxious and tense. You can often remember them in detail. This can have more to do with the Heart than with the Liver.

Traditional herbal and acupuncture point formulas to treat sleep will often treat the Heart as well. Insomnia and/or dream disturbances are the first symptom of Heart dysfunction which a patient notices.

The Heart loathes heat

Though the Heart is a yin organ, it is very yang in nature - it's element is fire and it is related to summer. Both the Heart and Liver (which also has a fire type association – more later on that) can have yang disorders such as deficiency of Heart yang, or Liver yang rising. An excess affecting the Heart is Heart fire. More heat is always a Heart excess and if the client is has it, they will have an aversion to heat and probably a thirst for cold drinks.

External pathogens attack the Pericardium *first*, rather than attacking the Heart directly. A biomedical example of this is pericarditis – an infection/inflammation condition of the body that eventually attacks the pericardial sac.

The Heart controls speech

Remember the connection of the Heart with Shen and the tongue. If one is very talkative, this can indicate an excessive condition of the Heart. If one has aphasia, this can indicate Heart Blood stagnation. Stuttering is also a heart disorder. Speech related to psychological disorders such as incoherent or wild crazy speech can also be Heart and Shen related.

THE HEART CHANNEL

The Heart channel or Heart meridian originates in the Heart organ, emerges from it and goes through the breathing diaphragm, connects to the Small Intestine, then branches out to the throat and the eye. Another branch of the Heart Channel enters the Lungs, emerging at the axilla (armpit) and joins the superficial channel running along the medial aspect of the arm and ends at the tip of the little finger.

SMALL INTESTINE

The Small Intestine is related to and paired with the Heart. The Small Intestines channel connects to the Heart channel and both are Fire organs per the Five Element Theory. Know the two functions of the Small Intestine below.
1. Small Intestine organ controls the receiving and transportation of digested food
2. The Small Intestine separates fluids, dividing the pure from the turbid/impure

Control receiving and transportation of digested food
The Stomach receives food. It grinds up the food and drink (or as the *Neijing* puts it, ripens and rots food and drink), then passes it on to the Small Intestine. The Small Intestine's job is to separate the useful or pure nutrients from the turbid (not so pure) matter. The turbid matter is discarded as waste with the solid turbid matter going to the Large Intestine and the liquid turbid matter going to the Kidney and Bladder.

The Small Intestine separates fluids
Basically as described in the paragraph above. But you still need to know the two functions.

SMALL INTESTINE'S RELATIONSHIP TO THE HEART

The movement/transportation of fluids is the job of the Small Intestine. Purer, cleaner parts of food are used and absorbed by the body while the turbid stuff is excreted. A dysfunction of the Small

Intestine results in an inability to separate that which is useful (pure) from that which is waste (impure/dirty/turbid). The two will very likely mix together resulting in diarrhea with undigested food in it. Traditionally in Chinese medicine, one promotes urination in order to stop diarrhea.

The Small Intestine has more to do with **heat** than with anything else. Pathologically, heat in the Heart can cause diarrhea. Heat in the Heart can come from over-thinking, anxiety and worry. Heat in the Heart, can manifest on the tip of the tongue as redness, as well as ulcers or blisters on the tongue and as jitteriness or anxiousness.

Heat can also be *transmitted* from the Heart to the Small Intestine. Because the Small Intestine sends fluids to the Urinary Bladder where it becomes urine, this heat is also passed along to the Bladder and manifests as urgent need to urinate, painful urination and dark urine. The urine may be scanty when this happens and it may burn when the bladder is voided. These all look like UTI symptoms. Patients who go to the doctor with UTI symptoms but who test negative for bacterial infection are probably experiencing Heart heat transferred to the Small Intestine and then on to the Bladder.

This page intentionally left blank

CHAPTER 6
Liver and Gallbladder

The Liver is regarded as the most important organ in Chinese medicine in terms of women's health. (In case you're wondering, for men it's the Kidney.) I'm not suggesting men can't have Liver dysfunction too – they can. But most women have some variety of Liver dysfunction with endocrine/hormonal problems. When the endocrine/hormonal problems are in excess, treat the Liver; when they are deficient, treat the Kidney.

Location

From a Western medicine perspective, the liver is located on the right side of the body below the right side of the rib cage. In Chinese medical anatomy, the Liver is still located on the right side of the body within the *Middle* Jiao.

However, the function of the Liver is said to be *Lower* Jiao. The Liver *channel/meridian* begins on the big toe on the lateral side of the corner of the toenail.

> When you study pulse diagnosis, however, the Liver pulse is felt in the middle position on the left arm. Why? Lots of guesses from various practitioners and interpreters of Chinese medical literature.
>
> The most important thing to remember is from Chapter 16 of the Nanjing, which says there are many ways to take pulses. Pick the one that works for you and verify your diagnosis by looking at all of the signs and symptoms.

Constitution

Constitutionally, the Liver has both Yin and Yang properties.

Yin

I mentioned a chapter or two ago that Yin and Blood are closely related. Yin is substantive and moist, Blood is also substantive and liquid. Both provide foundations/substance for the body. So the Yin of the Liver is closely related to the Blood of the Liver. You will frequently hear the term Liver Blood. When you hear this term the practitioner or teacher is also talking about the Liver Yin.

Yang

Yang and Qi (like Yin and Blood) are also closely related. Yang is functional and active, Qi is light and active also and is thus an expression of Yang. Another term you will hear frequently in Chinese medicine is Liver Qi. This is the function of the liver and is the energy expressed in the Lower Jiao. In women you will see this most obviously in menstrual dysfunction. Cramping, spotting, and clotting during menses are all related to dysfunction of the Liver Qi.

FUNCTIONS OF THE LIVER

Always memorize the functions of an organ. In addition to knowing the main functions for the Liver, you also need to know the sub functions. I think the best way to summarize this for you is in a table. *Memorize the whole table.* We'll talk about it in more detail below.

Main Liver function	Subfunction/s to know
Liver stores Blood	Regulates Blood volume in relation to rest and activity
	Regulates menstruation
	Moistens and nourishes the eyes and the sinews/tendons
	Liver is in charge of the biorhythms
Liver ensures the smooth flow of Qi	Governs the flow of Qi
	Affects the emotional state
	Affects digestion
	Affects secretion of bile

The Liver stores Blood

This was one of the harder concepts to wrap my mind around. In biomedicine blood isn't stored, but circulates. In the years I've been practicing and studying I've come to think that it is the essence contained in the blood that is banked. The Liver, for instance, really does "store" blood in the night, converting blood sugars into longer term storage. If you think of it like that, the uterus does too, storing blood as uterine lining. I don't know if thinking like this will help you, but I offer it up to you nonetheless.

The Liver stores blood, but is not the only organ to do so: Uterus and Chong (Penetrating) Vessel do also. But because Liver stores blood, it is able to regulate menstruation, regulate the bio-clock, and to house the Hun or Ethereal Soul (see the last page of this chapter for more on that one).

There are several sub-functions of storing Blood you need to know as well.

The Liver regulates Blood volume in relation to rest and activity.

When the body rests at night the blood goes to the Liver: circulation is slower and the body gets cooler as a result. In the morning as soon as your eyes open from sleep the Blood begins to circulate more fully again throughout the body. When you work during the day your body needs this blood in order to function.

The Liver regulates menstruation

The Liver is designed to control the smooth graceful accumulation and circulation of energy or Qi. I think of it as a benevolent traffic cop or air traffic controller. In some Chinese literature it is compared to a General controlling the movement of the troops. When all is going well, the energy flow is smooth and the emotions are balanced.

When you see a person who is very quick to anger, flies off the handle easily, is irritable, a woman who has signs of PMS, clots when she menstruates, a person who is depressed, and/or who cries easily, you are looking at what is often referred to as "Liver Qi Stagnation." That means the Liver is not able to smoothly move the Qi through the body so it gets 'stuck' in various places.

You'll see a person sigh a lot for no reason or they will talk about clotting in their menstrual bloods when you ask them about that. These are signs of 'stuck' Liver Qi. The sighing is a way to release the Qi that gets stuck in the chest. The clotting is because the Qi isn't moving well, so the Blood (which is moved *by* the Qi) is getting stuck and coagulating.

> I've noticed that smokers don't seem to have this sighing thing quite as bad even when they do have Liver Qi stagnation. Why? I think it's because the deep inhales and exhales involved in smoking are temporarily keeping the Qi moving in the chest. I'm not implying this is healthy! I'm just noticing. You'd get far better benefits by stepping outside away from the smoking area and doing breath work!

The Liver moistens and nourishes the eyes and the sinews.

Look back at the Five Element correspondence chart. When a person is Liver Blood deficient, the symptoms are dryness and an inability to move the moisture around the body. Symptoms include dry eyes and tight tendons. In TCM eye diseases are often treated by focusing on the Liver.

> Fun fact: computer screens and televisions negatively impact the condition of your Liver Blood. I have sat in front of this danged screen for more years than I want to admit and have had chronic dry eye problems, despite the herbs and nutritional therapy I treat myself with. It wasn't until I went on vacation in the middle of nowhere for a couple of weeks, promptly lost my phone, and discovered I had no internet connection for my laptop that I realized how strongly my screen addiction was impacting my Liver Blood. All of my dry eye problems disappeared within a week because there was no reason to look at a screen. That was a wake-up call.

Applying that to patients, you have to know that many times they are coming to you for band-aid fixes for their bad lifestyle habits. Just good to know.

Convulsions, tremors, and muscle cramps are all tendon/sinew conditions. These are all conditions of Wind, be that internal wind or external wind. Wind, again, is associated with the Liver and with wood in the Five Element chart. Wind moves, shakes the limbs of trees, is fast and unpredictable. Shaking and moving symptoms are *always* Wind related in TCM. It helps to think of our limbs as tree limbs. ☺

The Liver is in charge of the biorhythms.
Liver controls the biorhythms of the body by controlling the circulation of Qi. Qi cycles through the 12 regular channels over and over again in this pattern:

Lung → Large Intestine → Stomach → Spleen → Heart → Small Intestine → Bladder → Kidney → Pericardium → San Jiao → Gallbladder → Liver.

Once the end of the cycle is reached, it repeats with Liver passing back to Lung and so on for ever and ever amen…or until you die….whichever comes first. Energy switches from one channel the next every 2 hours or so. The Liver hours are from 1am – 3am and from 1pm – 3pm.

Fun thing to do: If you have a tendency to wake in the middle of the night, make note of the time period and take a peek at a chart of the various times associated with the channels.

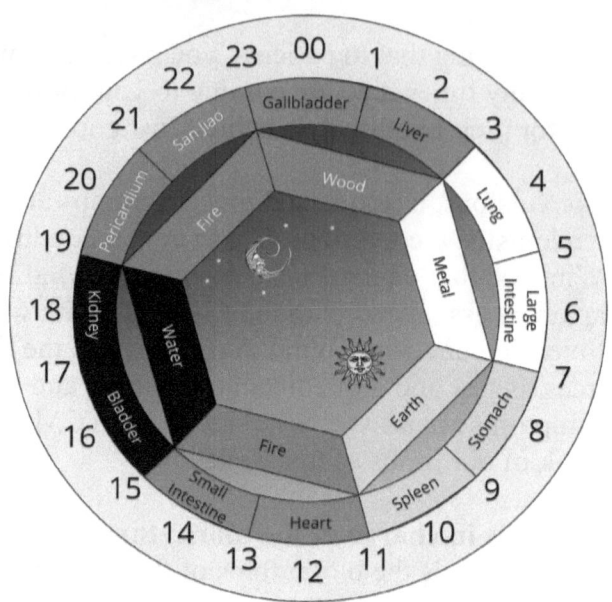

Liver ensures the smooth flow of Qi.

Because Liver does is in charge of Qi flow through the body it also governs emotions, digestion and the secretion of bile.

Governs the flow of Qi

There is Qi for each organ of the body. The action of Spleen Qi is to rise upward. Stomach Qi descends. Lung Qi disperses upward, outward, and downward. Large Intestine Qi descends. All of these rely on the regulating Qi of the Liver to keep them moving correctly.

Affects the emotional state

Emotional disorders, especially those of temper, depression, distress, irritability, PMS, and frustration are closely related to the Liver. When the Liver qi is obstructed there is distress and anger. When the Liver qi is congested there is irritability, PMS.

Affects digestion

While it is true that the Spleen and Stomach control digestion (a Middle Jiao function), their Qi cannot move freely if the Qi of the Liver is congested. Congested is another way to say blocked or stagnant. When the Liver Qi is not free to flow (which can occur as a result of worry, stress, anger and more), the Wood element will then overact or overcontrol the Earth element – Spleen and Stomach. That's straight up Five Element theory, yo!

> Cat's note: not *all* emotional disorders are related to Liver. TCM is just not that cut and dried.
>
> You must take all factors into consideration before diagnosing a problem as Liver related just because it is an emotional dysfunction. Mania, for example, is usually related to the Heart, sadness and grief to the Lungs, fear to the Kidneys. Don't get sucked into believing that all emotions flow from the Liver!
>
> This is a common mistake many people new to TCM make. You'll get lots more on this in Energetics, Point Locations, Diagnostics, Treatment of Disease classes and so on, so don't think you have to memorize all of this right this second. Just bear this principle in mind.

"Liver Overacting on Spleen" is actually a pretty common diagnosis in clinic. This is a person with a Liver problem which will then have an effect on Spleen Qi. Spleen Qi then can't ascend which can result in loose stools, diarrhea, gas, bloating, or even constipation (when the Spleen Qi is so weak it can't push waste out).

"Liver Overacting on Stomach" is the Liver energy impacting the Stomach Qi, making it hard for the Stomach to do it's job of making food descend. Symptomatically that looks like an uncomfortable sensation of food just sitting in the stomach (called "food stagnation") and maybe even visible bloating right around the stomach area (called "focal distention"). That patient might have hiccups or vomiting.

Affects secretion of bile
When the Liver Qi is full, it is transferred to the Gallbladder where the Qi is stored and transformed into bile.

Bonus fun things to know about the Liver

- Sinews:
are nourished by Liver Blood

- Nails:
are byproducts and offshoots of the sinews. When Liver blood is deficient the nails will be pale. They can also be unnourished causing brittle nails or nails that split in layers. You can also see nail ridges which run either horizontally or vertically or both.

- Eyes:
Liver Qi goes to the eyes. If the eyes are dry or if there are floaters in the vision it indicates Liver dysfunction. Floaters are those little bits that people see in their field of vision when they are looking at a clear blue sky or a white wall. There's nothing on the wall or in the sky, but rather are in the vision itself.

- Ethereal soul:
The Ethereal soul is yang in nature and is rooted in the Liver when there is adequate Liver blood. Inadequate Blood causes the soul is unrooted, disturbed and restless. Can result in sleep, talking in one's sleep and that dream disturbed sleep thing we spoke of earlier.

(Again, don't get the idea that dream disturbed sleep is always related to Liver…it's often related to Heart dysfunction in TCM. Remember: no hard and fast rules! Every condition, every patient is a unique combination which you will come to recognize more easily than you think.)

- Anger:
  Distress, depression, frustration, and anger are often related to Liver.

- The Liver controls planning and acts as a "general." (And it gets pretty pissed off when things don't go like it wants!)

GALLBLADDER

Functions:
1. Stores and secretes Bile
   This is like it's biomedical function. The Liver creates bile, passes it to the Gallbladder through the common bile duct. The Gallbladder stores it and concentrates it then releases the bile into the Small Intestine as needed to help digest fats. Actually, the Gallbladder is the only yang organ that doesn't deal *directly* with food.

   All Gallbladder problems involve digestive disorders and there is close relationship between the Small Intestine and the Gallbladder and digestion.

2. The Gallbladder controls Decisiveness
   While the Liver controls planning, the Gallbladder controls one's ability to be decisive. In Chinese if you say someone has a "big gallbladder" you are saying that they are very brave, decisive and fast in decision making. The term for this is "Dan Da." The opposite of this descriptive is "Dan Xiao" or "small gallbladder" meaning one is timid, fluctuates in his/her decisions and has trouble deciding.

3. Controls Sinews
   Like Liver, Gallbladder controls sinews. Liver blood *nourishes* the sinews, but the Gallbladder provides qi to the sinews to assure movement and agility. When you study the Gallbladder channel in Energetics 3 you will see that the channel has many points on it that can assist the smooth movement of sinews. You might also notice that where the Gallbladder channel flows down the leg it passes right down

the fascia latte on the lateral side of the thigh as well as through may other fibrous fascia coverings of the body.

As a matter of fact, Gallbladder 34 is the control or convergent point for the sinews of the whole body. It's on the lateral side of the lower leg not too far from Stomach 36 (some books say it is 1 cun posterior/lateral to ST 36).

Relationship between Liver and Gallbladder

Liver creates bile and sends it to the Gallbladder which stores, concentrates, and secretes bile. They are dependent upon each other, especially in their relationship via Qi (because Liver Qi drives the other organ Qi's). Together, the Liver and Gallbladder are responsible for the smooth flow of Qi. They are also critical to one's ability to get things done on the planet: Liver gives you the ability to plan while Gallbladder gives you the ability to be decisive and get busy.

All Gallbladder problems are treated through treating the Liver.

The sides of the tongue reflect the health or dysfunction of the Liver and Gallbladder.

CHAPTER 7
Lung and Large Intestine

Earlier in this tome, the wordiest-Cliff-Notes-ever version of Chinese medicine foundations, I said that the Chinese were big on rank and function in society. Once upon a time the organs weren't referred to as merely organs, but had rank and a function in the society of the body. The Heart is the Emperor, the Liver is the General, and the Lungs? They are the Prime Minister to the Emperor. Sometimes they are called "the coach roof" meaning they cover and protect the Heart as the 2nd in command should do.

Though that seems like a pretty badass role in life, the Lungs are considered to be delicate organs in Chinese medicine. Why? Because they are the most external of the Yin organs, the ones that have first contact with the outside world. There is nowhere else in the body that a Yin organ has such intimate contact with the outside environment with all of its' pollutants and microorganisms. The Lungs are our first line of defense.

Location
The Lungs are the highest Yin organs in the body. According to Chinese anatomical thought, the Lung is located in the chest, moreso on the right than the left. And indeed, in western medicine you will learn that the right lung has three lobes while the left lung has only two and is slightly smaller to make room for the Heart.

In the invasion of the six external pathogens, the Lung is generally the first to be affected due to its close interaction with the outside world by drawing in external air. Note that when you catch a cold, first the nose is affected (which is associated with the Lung), then the throat, then tonsils or bronchials.

The Lung Channel
The Lung channel whose formal name is "The Lung Meridian of the Hand Taiyin," originates in the *Middle Jiao*

at about the Ren 12 point (draw a line from your umbilicus to the sternal costal angle – you'll find Ren 12 in the middle of this line). From here the meridian goes downward to connect to the Large Intestine and then does a U-turn, going up through the Stomach and diaphragm before going to the Lung. It ascends through the throat with a branch off of the channel going to the lateral chest and then down to the upper extremities.

Per the Five Elements, the element of earth generates metal (which is the elemental association for Lung). From a Five Element treatment perspective, if you want to tonify the Lung Qi, tonify the Stomach and the Spleen.

FUNCTIONS OF THE LUNG

There are several functions and sub-functions of the Lung you need to know. Memorize the chart below and then we'll get into more detail about each function in the text below. Not all of the main funcitons have sub functions to know.

Main Function of Lung	Sub-function/s to know
Governs Respiration	*No sub functions to know*
Governs Qi	Transformation of Qi occurs through control of respiration
	Transportation/movement of Qi
Controls channels and blood vessels	*No sub functions to know*
Governs dispersing	Dispersing – outward movemet
Governs descending	Fresh air downward to Dantian
	Descends Body Fluids to the Bladder
	Descends wastes to the Lower Jiao
Regulates water passage	Lung is the upper source of water in the body (i.e., water in the Upper Jiao)
Lung opens to the nose	*No sub functions to know*
Houses the Corporeal Soul, the Po	

The Lung Governs Qi and Respiration
Respiration
The Lungs are the origin for the exchange of Qi with the outside world - inhaling and exhaling. Lungs filter the air, while the Liver filters blood and the Kidney filters water. You exhale exhausted Qi through both your Lungs and through your sweat.

At birth a baby's first action is to inhale, taking in Qi from the air and descending it downward into the Lungs. Lung qi by nature descends outward and downward. You can see the outward action when you inhale deeply and your chest expands outward. You can see the downward action by inhaling deeply and slowly and feeling the abdomen get larger as the air goes downward. When this movement is impaired, like when Lung Qi ascends too much, there is asthma, wheezing, coughing and more.

Qi
Transformation of Qi occurs through the control of respiration.
The *Neijing* says the universe feeds human beings from heaven (air) and earth (food). There is one further source of energy for humans and that is the Qi you get from your parents at birth. That's kind of a starter pack – happy birthday from mom and dad.
- Da Qi or Big Qi – fresh air.
- Food Qi or Gu Qi – vital qi you get from your food and drink.
- Primary Qi – that's the starter pack you get at birth from your parents.

Transportation of Qi
This is the movement of Qi. This includes the ascending and descending of qi. When you inhale, qi descends; when you exhale, qi ascends.

When the Lung Qi is weak (a Lung Qi deficiency), the signs and symptoms show as a pale face, shortness of breath, soft/small/weak voice, and fatigue. Disorders in the transportation of Lung Qi include tightness in the chest, dyspnea (difficult breathing), wheezing and cough.

The Lung Controls Channels and Blood Vessels

The Heart and Lung make up the pulmonary circulation. In Chinese medicine the Lung is above all other organs. *All* vertical channels pass through the Lung. The *Neijing* says "the Lung meets with all channels and collaterals." Another quote from the *Neijing*: "Lung controls the Hundred Channels."

Why is this significant? Three reasons.
1. Pulse diagnosis. The Lung channel runs through the places on the wrist where you feel for the pulse in diagnosis. Because the Lung controls all channels and vessels you can feel excesses and deficiencies through the lung pulse.

2. Lung is beneficial for energy and blood flow. Blood flow is related to breath. We even count pulse versus breath and in Chinese medicine normal pulse/breath is 4 beats of the heart for one inhale. 6+ beats of the pulse per breath is considered to be a fast pulse and reflects a condition of heat in the body.

3. Blood flow will come like waves corresponding with the breath. Lung sends blood to the peripheral areas of the body along with the energy of the Heart. (And because of this you can sometimes sense what feels like an irregularity in the pulse that is really the breath affecting the pulse.)

Governs dispersing and descending

Lung Qi disperses outward and descends downward.

Dispersing

The sweat pores (all 36,000 or so of them) open when you inhale so they can let wastes out. When you exhale, the pores close, holding the Qi in. Lung Qi sends vital substances to the superficial areas.

It sends Wei Qi to the superficial areas of the body to aid in defense. Your Lungs and skin are your first layers of defense. Indeed, the Lungs and skin are considered part of the same system. When the Wei Qi is healthy, the pores open to release wastes, cleanse the body, and maintain water metabolism. When you exhale Wei Qi closes the pores to protect the interior. If the Wei Qi is deficient, the pores cannot be closed properly, immunity is lowered, and one is more vulnerable to invasion by the external evils.

I think of this deficient Wei Qi state kind of like a window that doesn't seal or has a broken pane. It lets rain and wind in when it should be keeping them out.

Lung also disperses Body Fluids to the skin to keep the skin moist and supple.

Descending
Descends Qi Downward
Qi in the Lung disperses in all directions, but the *descending function* is especially important. Lung Qi descends fresh air downward to the Dantian where it meets with Gu (Food) Qi.

> OK, what? The Dantian is an area just below the belly button and in the center of the body. In Qigong and in Daoist practices you focus on this area and visualize the Qi of the universe flowing into it. Another name for the Dantian is the "red elixir field" or "the fields of cinnabar." Cinnabar is also called mercury. Mercury in Chinese medical history could either be an amazing medicine when prepared properly or it could be an intense poison in the hands of someone who had no clue what they were doing. The Dantian is like that too – if

you refine your energy it is the source of great power and love. If you don't it can kill you.

If you want to know more, read *In Search of the Medicine Buddha* on your next break from school. Really good read.

Asthma patients are often shallow breathers, breathing into the upper chest only and unable to get the breath to descend to the Dantian. By the way, this totally tracks with biomedicine. There is a lower diaphragm associated with the pelvic floor. When you inhale the breathing diaphragm lowers and so does the diaphragm in the pelvic region. If the pelvic floor is too tight, that lower diaphragm doesn't descend properly on the inhale and the breath will be shallow.

The descending function also assists in the production and transport of Body Fluids. It works like this:

You eat and drink, which goes first to the Stomach. The Stomach grinds up the food and drink and passes it to the Small Intestine which separates the good stuff (pure) from the bad stuff (turbid). Turbid fluids go the Urinary Bladder. Pure fluids are transferred to the Spleen. Solid turbid stuff goes to the Large Intestine. The liquids that are reusable in the Large Intestine are reabsorbed and transferred to the Spleen.

What does the Spleen do with all that fluid? Transforms it into Body Fluids and into Blood. It sends some to the Lung to disperse and moisten the tissues, sends some to the Heart to transform into Blood.

This is a Dr Qianzhi Wu diagram. Took me years to really wrap my head round it, but you might be a smarter person than I am!

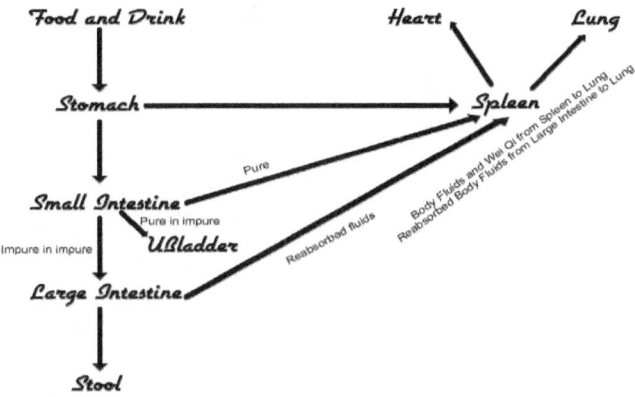

Descends wastes to the Lower Jiao
The Lower Jiao is designed to channel out wastes. In order for the Lung to maintain good condition it cannot tolerate foreign bodies. Excreting this waste helps the Lung maintain health.

> Know: The Lung's descending function sends air, Body Fluids, and wastes downward.

The Lung regulates water passage

Remember the thing I said earlier about the San Jiao (aka Triple Warmer or Triple Burner) being like a water transport system? Think of it kind of like a three-tiered fountain with a pump dispersing the water between the three tiers.

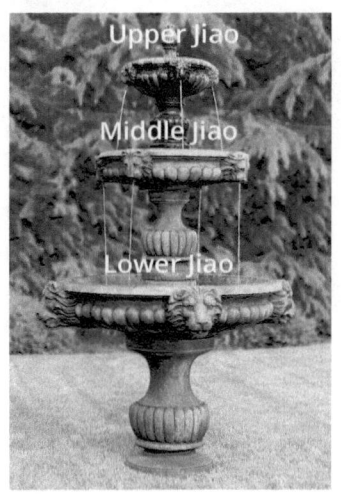

The Lung is the upper *source* of water in the body – the source for the Upper Jiao. It moves the water in the upper body. The Middle Jiao through which water is passed is the Spleen/Stomach and the Lower Jiao or water passage is the Urinary Bladder and Kidney.

Water passage is regulated between these 3 Jiao through the dispersing and descending functions of the Lung. This maintains proper water balance in all parts of the body.

When you exhale, waste in the form of carbon dioxide exits the body through the nose and mouth. So do extra Body Fluids in the form of vapor. Wastes also exit the body via liquid waste sent to the Bladder.

This changes seasonally. In the summer the body sweats more, releasing more body fluids out through the sweating pores and less through the Bladder. In the winter, when the universal energy is down, less fluid is dispersed through the skin and more to the urinary bladder.

The Lungs are sensitive to the season and to temperature changes. It is the most important organ to communicate with the outside world and regulates water balance through the dispersal and descending function. While fluid is *generated* by the Spleen, Stomach, Small and Large Intestines, the Lung remains the upper *source* of water in the body. This does not refer to the generation of fluid, but to the lung's ability to disperse and descend fluids. If this function is not working properly there can be water retention in the Lung (pulmonary edema), puffy eyes, and facial edema.

Lung opens to the nose

The color of the nose, quality and quantity of nasal discharge, nosebleeds, and more all reflect the condition of the Lung. Symptoms of the nose are very important for diagnosis of Lung problems. Examples:
- Watery loose discharge from the nose can indicate invasion of wind and cold.

- Sticky, yellow/green discharge can indicate heat in the Lung, infection or inflammation.

- Nasal bleeding or bloody sputum can indicate toxic heat.

    Note: nose bleeds when one is *not* sick can indicate something other than a Lung dysfunction, such as a very strong Yang constitution, the ingestion of an awful lot of Yang stuff, and very high blood pressure.

    Seriously on the blood pressure. Use points to stop the bleeding, but definitely check the pressure. I saw this recently and it was a little humbling to learn I wasn't treating what I thought I was (epistaxis due to an internal dry heat and extreme yin deficiency – which she did have), but a dangerously high blood pressure. Learned *that* lesson!

- Stuffy nose with no discharge and impaired sense of smell can reflect stagnant Lung qi.

Lung controls the skin and hair growing from the skin

The skin to Lung relationship has to do with the dispersing function. There is a form of asthma often triggered by allergies which is associated with dermatitis and eczema. This condition reflects either heat in the body that was generated from within or exterior heat that has permeated deep in the body. When this form of asthma is worse, the skin is often better – when the asthma is less problematic the dermatitis is often worse. This is because the Lung must disperse the heat somehow, either through the Lungs or through the skin.

Dry skin is usually associated with Lung also. The Wei qi, which is part of the Lung qi, opens and closes sweat pores. When the Wei qi is weak it cannot close those pores again, which can dry the skin.

Dry skin can also be associated with Heart. The Heart provides the material foundation of sweat (Blood, in case you are pondering, is the foundation of sweat). When there is a Heart Blood deficiency some of the symptoms can be dermatitis and dry skin because the Heart is unable to spare enough "juice" to make sweat.

The Lung houses the Corporeal Soul or the Po

Po in Chinese can be translated as "White Ghost." It is said when the Lung Qi is weak one will dream of white objects. The Po can be damaged by trauma, emotional shock or grief. Asthma, especially adult-onset asthma, is often due to childhood abuse and/or a improper nutritional support during childhood.

Dreams

You can sometimes diagnose Lung problems through dreams. In general, if you dream you get a gift, then the body is in a weakened condition – you need the gift. If you dream of white objects, bloody dreams, or killing, the Lungs are deficient. If you dream you *give* a gift, this may indicate an excess condition. When the Lungs are in excess you may also dream of weeping. If you have a repeat dream, you are in need of whatever it is that is repeating.

Sayings regarding Lung

- The Lungs control the 100 (Blood) vessels
  There is a strong connection between the Lung and Heart. In Chinese medicine Lung 9 on the medial wrist is *the* big influential point for blood vessels. You see this intimate connection between the two organs in biomedicine too. A heart problem often generates a lung problem and vice versa. Bronchitis over time progresses from acute episodes to chronic bronchitis, to emphysema, and then to pulmonary heart disease like COPD. The exchange of blood between these two organs is so immediate and intimately connected that one cannot be affected without

affecting the other.

- Lung loathes Cold.
  Lung is sensitive to weather changes and any temperature changes. When the weather turns cold you feel it in your lungs and get goose bumps on your skin.

- Lung controls the voice
  Zhong qi is the "gathering qi" or the collective qi of the chest encompassing the heart and Lung qi. Its' health or lack thereof controls the voice when Zhong qi is transformed into voice.

- Lungs are located on the right or descending side.
  OK, really they're located on both sides, but you can detect Lung Qi most easily on the right. The right hand pulse is where you feel Lung health or dysfunction, for example.
  The qi of the body ascends on the left (controlled by the Liver) and descends on the right (controlled by the Lungs).

LARGE INTESTINE

Functions
1. Receive digested food from the Stomach and Small Intestine
2. Reabsorb body fluids and send them to the Spleen
3. Move the bowels (descending qi again) and get rid of the stool.
   When the stool is loose, not enough has been absorbed; when there is constipation too much has been absorbed.

RELATIONSHIP BETWEEN LUNG AND LARGE INTESTINE

The descending function of the Lung Qi helps bowel movements. The Large Intestine resorbs bodily fluids to help moisten the Lung.

You can sometimes treat asthma and lung function by promoting bowel movements. Xuan Bai Chen Qi Tang is a formula which promotes the descending Lung Qi function and assists with this problem within 2-3 weeks.

CHAPTER 8
Spleen and Stomach

One of the many things you will hear about the Spleen is that it is the Root of Post-heaven Qi. That means that other than breathing, what we eat and drink and the quality of that input is responsible for all of the Qi we are able to generate ourselves. Pre-heaven Qi is the "trust fund" or starter pack our parents give us when we are conceived and developed.

Spleen is closely tied to the Stomach in a Yin and Yang relationship. Remember the Yin and Yang Principles?

- **Opposition.**
  The Spleen Qi ascends while the Stomach Qi descends.

- **Interdependence.** One *has* to have the other in order to function.

- **Mutual Consumption.** One feeds the other.

- **Inter-transformation.** One feeds and is fed by the other. The energy of the one is transformed into the energy of the other.

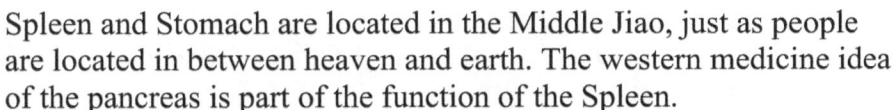

Spleen and Stomach are located in the Middle Jiao, just as people are located in between heaven and earth. The western medicine idea of the pancreas is part of the function of the Spleen.

FUNCTIONS OF THE SPLEEN

There are nine functions of the Spleen you need to memorize. OK, the last one isn't a function, but know it anyhow. As usual, we'll get to the specifics in the following paragraphs.

1. Spleen governs transformation and transportation
2. Controls the ascending of Qi
3. Raises clear Yang
4. Controls Blood

5. Controls the muscles and four limbs
6. Houses the intellect and thoughts
7. Is the root of Post-heaven Qi
8. Origin of birth and development
9. Spleen *dislikes* cold and has an *aversion* to damp

Govern transformation and transportation

This is the main function of the Spleen. It is the Stomach that holds, ripens and rots food and drink, but is it the Spleen which transforms it into Food (Gu) Qi.

There are 2 kinds of Qi derived from food:
1. **Ying Qi or Nutritive Qi**.
   Ying Qi is transported to the heart and trasformed into Blood. When one has a poor appetite and no Ying Qi is available for Heart blood, one will often have palpitations and a poor memory as a result.

2. **Wei Qi or Defensive Qi**
   Wei Qi is transported to the Lung to be dispersed to the skin, the outer protective layer. When you sleep at night, the Wei Qi also sleeps, going inward. This is why you tend to get colder at night and cover up to protect your internal organs.

The Spleen also regulates the digestion and use of Water, which is lifted upward to the Lungs then to the surface of the body as sweat.

If the Spleen cannot raise the water and Food Qi upward then there is a condition of dampness or food stagnation. The substance of the Spleen is the Food Qi generated. The raising force of the Spleen is its Yang function.

A Spleen deficiency will also lead to a Blood deficiency since the substances needed are not available for building blood. It also leads to immune deficiency since there is no production of Wei Qi.

Remember that the Spleen is the *middle* source of water in the body, but does not store water. The Lungs are the upper source and the Kidneys are the lower source.

Controls the Ascending of Qi

A primary function of the Spleen is to raise or lift and thus raise and hold the organs in place. A Spleen deficiency weakens this lifting function organ. When it becomes a severe deficiency, organs can prolapse or fall out of place. Uterine, bladder, stomach, and rectal prolapse are all very real possibilities. From a Western medicine perspective this happens when internal musculature cannot hold up the organs. Remember that one of the Spleen's funcitons is to control the muscles and the four limbs. More on that in a minute.

Without the ascending of Qi, lower digestive functions can also be impaired. Diarrhea and loose or unformed stools are possible outcomes. . . pardon the pun.

Raising Clear Yang upwards

Clear Yang is Yang Qi that is not turbid or 'polluted.' Qi is very light and ascends upward to the head which is nourished and supported by the Yang resulting in clearer thinking. You could legitimately think of this as part of the ascending of Qi function we just talked about, since Qi and Yang are so closely tied together.

Controls Blood

There are two major ways in which the Spleen controls Blood.

First, it produces Ying or Nutritive Qi by extracting the good stuff from the food and drink you take in. The Ying Qi is then supplied to the Heart, which uses it to produce Blood. Similar in biomedicine – nutrient extraction which then flows through the Blood to feed the body.

The Spleen Qi also controls Blood by helping to hold it inside the vessels. Conditions of bleeding such as uterine breakthrough bleeding (not the normal menstrual bleeding) and bleeding gums, can be caused by insufficient Spleen Qi.

Controls the muscles and the four limbs

Muscles will be weak or atrophy if the Spleen Qi is weak. Why? Because the Spleen, the "Storehouse of Grains" as it is sometimes called, supplies the nutrients the body needs. Poor nutrients = weak muscles. Nutrition matters!

Spleen houses the intellect and thoughts.

Thoughts and memory are part of the Spleen's function. It influences our capacity for thinking, studying, concentration, memorization for work and school. This is part of the Ascending Qi and Ascending Pure Yang functions of the Spleen.

Additionally, the Heart houses the Mind (one way to think of Shen). If you want to memorize and think, you *need* good quality Blood, which the Spleen controls. Some writings say the Shen is rooted in the blood – like it's the *home* of the Shen. You need a place for your Shen to rest in order for it to help you through school.

Remember too that the Heart is responsible for *short term memory*. The Kidney is responsible for *long* term memory. So if you are studying for a test, you need the Heart to help you remember the material and spit it back out in a manner that gets you a passing grade. BUT, if you really want to know and integrate what you are learning, you also need a happy healthy Kidney to help you retain it. You nourish your brain function by nourishing the Marrow – that that's about making your Spleen, Heart, and Kidney delightfully happy.

And I'll be honest with you: that's really hard to do while you're studying your buns off in school. Takes a lot of diligence and I did a crappy job of it!

Spleen is the root of Post Heaven Qi.

We've touched on this a bit, but here's a quick review. When you are conceived, your parents are the ones supplying your Qi. When you are in utero, it's your mother who supplies your Qi. This is referred to as pre-heaven Qi. When you are born, your first job is to take a breath. That's your first taste of *post-heaven* Qi. From then until you die, inhaling and exhaling (big Qi or da Qi) and eating and drinking (gu Qi) are your most common methods for acquiring more Qi.

Qigong practice is another form of acquiring Qi, even of acquiring Essence, but that's another discussion for later.

Origin of Birth and Development

Musculature and muscle development is controlled by the Spleen. If the Spleen is weak it cannot control the muscles or muscular development, impacting the health of the child approximately forever.

Spleen is dislikes Cold and has an aversion to Damp

Yeah, OK. Not really a function, but it's still a fact.

You need water - as a matter of fact, most of your body is made up of it. But you need it to be controlled in the body. It helps to think of your body like you would a garden. You can give the plants the "proper" amount of water, but if you have crappy drainage in your garden the roots of your plants will be waterlogged and unable to function properly.

So the same is true in your body. Too much water, or water not properly shuttled around the body, creates a condition called *dampness*. Dampness is extremely bad for the spleen. It creates swampy conditions in which the moisture doesn't move properly. That results in water retention in the wrong places. Water that doesn't flow correctly leads to phlegm – a sticky goo that can be created by dampness + either cold or heat. Cold congeals the damp into phlegm while heat cooks the damp down into phlegm. Either way, ick!

Another analogy comes from the 2 weeks I spent in Costa Rica in the rain forest. It was pretty, but so humid that it was hard to even take a short walk. One afternoon it was what should have been a pleasant 75 degrees Fahrenheit. The humidity was 100% and it wasn't raining. I made it about ¼ mile before I was too exhausted to continue. My clothes were stuck to my body, I was sweating profusely. Even trying to peel off my damp clothes when I dragged myself back to my cabin was even a huge chore.

So yeah. Damp in the body is like that. And it's super hard to resolve because it's so sticky. And it makes other things like conditions of Cold or Heat even more miserable because it kind of glues them in place. Yippee, right?

Wrapping it up, the Spleen *needs* warmth and dry in order to dry dampness.

STOMACH

Stomach functions to know

1. Spleen controls the receiving of food
   Stomach Qi holds ingested food so that the Stomach organ can ripen/rot it. The Stomach qi then descends, passing prepared foods on to the Small Intestine, so that the food does not stagnate. A rebellion or failure of Stomach Qi results in nausea, vomiting, hiccups.

2. Stomach rots and ripens the Food
   This is the *beginning* of digestion (...ok, technically, it starts in the mouth with chewing and salivary enzymes...). The rotting and ripening refers to the breakdown of food. The Spleen actually digests, extracting Food Qi from that which is rotted/ripened.

3. Stomach controls the transportation of food essence to the Spleen.
   So basically, it's not enough to ripen and rot, it's got to

deliver the goods to the Spleen.

4. Stomach controls descending of Qi
   Rotted and ripened food descends to the Small Intestine for nutrient extraction. Waste products descend to the Large Intestine/colon, rectum, and anus. All are downward moving. When the Qi cannot descend the waste the result is nausea, vomiting, and hiccups.

   Middle Jiao problems such as gas, bloating, diarrhea, nausea, vomiting and hiccups are widely seen in the clinic. You will learn more about this in later classes, but I'll tell you now that upper digestive dysfunction (nausea, vomiting and hiccups) are the result of Stomach dysfunction, while the lower stuff (gas, bloating, and diarrhea/loose stool) are the result of Spleen dysfunction

5. Stomach likes wetness and cold
   The Stomach, as a Yang organ, has a built-in dry/heat and doesn't want more! You will note that this is in direct opposition to the Spleen's preferences. This is why the diet and constitution must be balanced in order for the wheel to spin correctly!

   When you eat late at night both sleep and digestion are affected. The Stomach channel has one branch going to the Heart. When Stomach Qi is disturbed by a late meal it influences the Heart and can lead to dream disturbed sleep. In a nutshell, the fire of the digestion in the Stomach disturbs Shen.

   When the Stomach suffers from excess heat one of the symptomatic possibilities is toothache and/or bleeding gums, as there is part of the Stomach meridian that goes to the teeth and gums.

6. Dreams
   When one dreams of large meals the Stomach is deficient.
   When one dreams of hunger the Spleen is deficient.
   When one dreams of seeing the sun or of heaviness and

inability to move there is excess or damp heat in the body.

Relationship between Stomach and Spleen

Most engines work via a series of controlled explosions with cycles of intense energy and cycles of rest. As a matter of fact, things *move* because of a balance of opposites. The Spleen and Stomach are no exception. (OK, that's true for all of the Zangfu organ pairs, but we're only talking about this one right now.) The Yin and Yang pairing are opposing and complimentary properties and must remain in balance!

Look at the chart below and check out all of the oppositions that make the whole system work properly.

Spleen	Stomach
Yin	Yang
Qi ascends	Qi descends
If Qi does not ascend = diarrhea, gas bloating, loose stool	If Qi does not descend = nausea/vomit Hiccups
Likes dry/warm If the Spleen is too wet the Qi gets heavy and descends rather than rising. The result is diarrhea, gas, bloating, loose stool. The Spleen is already swampy, don't pour in more cold liquids/foods!	Likes cold/wet If the Stomach is too dry it cannot send the food downward to the Large Intestine. Dry and heat can lead to constipation. The Stomach is already a desert – don't start a fire!
Is easily prone to deficiency. Poor appetite, diarrhea/loose stool, poor memory and fatigue are indicators of this.	Is easily prone to excess and heat
Is prone to Yang deficiency. More cold and damp damages Spleen Yang.	Is prone to Yin deficiency. More heat damages the Yin of the Stomach.

If this happens the Yin becomes relatively too strong, extinguishing any fire present.	If this happens the Yang becomes relatively too strong

The Liver (Wood) can overact on the Spleen (Earth), attacking it and disturbing the original Qi causing the problems mentioned in the table above. When one doesn't eat well for a very long time the Liver becomes too strong and the middle Jiao (Spleen/Stomach) becomes too weak.

This page intentionally left blank

CHAPTER 9
The Kidney and Urinary Bladder

In Chinese medicine, the Kidneys are considered to be the Root of Life, the Root of Pre-heaven Qi and the Root of the Twelve Internal Organs. When you are born you get this 'trust fund' from your parents as well as Pre-heaven Essence is stored in the Kidneys. We'll get into what Essence is in the 2nd part of your Foundations education, but for now you just need to know that Essence, and all of the roots and pre-heavens are related to lifespan and longevity.

Location of the Kidney

In Chinese medical anatomy, the Kidneys are located in the lower abdominal area on both sides of the spine. In an 'intact' person there are two. You will see a couple of different 'versions' about where the Kidney is located in Chinese medical literature. These writings span a few thousand years, so values, philosophies, and the way the world and the body were viewed changed over time. This is why in some writings you will see that the author says the Kidney proper was located on the left side of the body while the kidney on the right side was the home of the *Mingmen* or the 'gate of vitality.' The Mingmen is where the fire of the Kidney originates – like an oven keeping the energy of the Kidney vital and moving. In later writings you will read that the right Kidney is the home of the Kidney Yin, the left is the home of the Kidney Yang, and in between the two is the Mingmen.

Don't get too 'fundamentalist' about any of this. Just take it in and breathe it out for now!

Kidney Channel/Meridian

The Kidney meridian is properly called "The Kidney Channel of the Foot Shaoyin." It connects to *all* other organs through its channel/meridian pathway... *except the Spleen*! More on that later.

The channel originates under the little toe, and passes through the sole of the foot obliquely to the navicular bone. It goes past the medial malleolus and along the posterior/medial line of the leg through the knee, entering the sacrum. It then enters the spine and travels through it until it reaches L2 (Du 4 point). At this point it goes out to the abdomen and connects to the Kidneys, then to the Urinary Bladder and to the Liver. It passes through the diaphragm, entering the Lungs, flowing up through the throat and ends at the root of the tongue. Again, on its path it connects to all organs *except the Spleen*.

Know these landmarks!

Origin – under little toe
⇩
Passes through the sole
of the foot obliquely
⇩
Navicular bone
⇩
Medial malleolus
⇩
Through knee
⇩
Sacrum
⇩
Enters Spine
⇩
Out to abdomen at L2 (Du 4)
⇩
Connects to the Kidneys
⇩
Urinary Bladder
⇩
Liver
⇩
Lungs -
There is a branch from the Lungs to the Heart
and a connection to the Pericardium Channel
⇩
Throat

⇩
Ends at root of tongue

By nature, Kidney Qi ascends, also going out and down. The upward motion is the most important to know, however.

Because the Kidney channel connects with the spine, the channel can treat problems of the sciatica as well as problems of the bones. The lower back is the residence of the Kidneys. Kidney problems can express as persistent pain in the lower back.

> Fun thing to know:
>
> If both the Kidneys and the lower back have pain in addition to burning urgent urination, you must refer a patient to a biomedical physician (MD) to test for Kidney infection. You will learn more about testing for this in your Physical Assessment classes, but this need for referral is especially true if there is pain upon *percussion*, which doesn't mean punching your patient in the kidney, but giving a firm tap on your own hand, which you cup over the kidneys. Don't try this without proper training!

Respiration is controlled by both the Lungs *and Kidneys*. Lung draws fresh air in and down to the Kidneys. The Kidneys control reception and retention of the breath. This is kind of a suction function, grabbing the inhaled breath so that the Qi can be extracted from the air. This is often referred to as Kidney grasping the breath or grasping the Lung Qi. When the Kidney is weak there can be shortness of breath and more difficulty inhaling than exhaling.

Wait a minute. . . why doesn't the Kidney connect to the Spleen? I'm just not ready to talk about that yet. Hang in there.

MAIN FUNCTIONS OF THE KIDNEY

Yay! More memorization! I've got 10 functions of the Kidney and a few sub-functions for you to know. Here they are in a fun table to memorize.

Main function of Kidney	Sub-functions to know
The Kidney stores essence, governs birth, growth, reproduction, and development	The Kidney stores essence • Congenital essence = prenatal or preheaven essence • Acquired essence = postnatal or postheaven essence
	The Kidney governs birth, growth, and development
	Kidney governs Reproduction
The Kidneys produce Marrow, fill up the Brain, and govern the Bones.	*(No sub-functions to memorize for these. Yay!)*
Kidney governs water by governing the opening and closing of the Urinary Bladder	
Kidney controls reception of Qi	
Kidney opens to the ears	
Kidney manifests on the hair	
Kidney opens the two lower orifices (anus, urethra/vagina)	
Kidney houses willpower	
The Kidneys are the Gate of Vitality or Ming Men	

All functions of the Kidney derive from the Kidney Qi (ok, actually, this is true of all organs). The Essence of the Kidney comes from your parents which is converted into Yuan or Primary Qi and then into Kidney Qi. When you talk about the Kidney, you're also talking about Kidney Essence, Kidney Qi, Kidney Yin, and Kidney Yang.

OK. Now that that's out of the way, let's explore the functions in more detail.

The Kidney stores essence, governs birth, growth, reproduction, and development

Let's break each one of those down a little more.

The Kidney stores essence

When an egg is fertilized in utero, the Essence supplied by the sperm is held by the woman who adds her own Essence to it to create new life. The combined Essence of both parents leads to new life.

There are two definitions of the Kidney in Chinese medicine:
- Narrow definition - a pair of literal organs
- Broad definition – the *external* kidneys (which consists of the penis, scrotum, and testes) and the *internal* kidneys consist of the kidney organ plus the prostate or the uterus. What about the *ovaries* in a female? Those fall under the Liver system in Chinese medicine.

Essence is *stored* in the Kidneys. That includes both the congenital essence (prenatal or pre-heaven essence), which one gets from the parents as described above, and the acquired essence (postnatal or post-heaven Essence - Da Qi and Gu Qi.

The quality and quantity of prenatal essence depends upon the parents' health and state of being at the time of conception. The Kidneys store most of their energy in the winter. This is the best time for conception and is the time when one can pass on the most and best energy/essence to the child

If the quality of the parents' health or their state of being was poor at the time of conception, poor essence or a lack of essence can be passed to the child from the parents. There is a "thing" in Chinese medicine about what are referred to as Saturday night babies – kids who were conceived after a night of partying. These kids can be 'essence challenged.' Chronically depressed patients might have had alcoholic parents, for example.

Diabetes, hypertension and such which are passed from the parents to the child through the genes reflects this. *If a patient comes to you with inherited or genetic problems, treat the Kidney.* The prognosis for an inherited disease like this is not as good as for an acquired infectious disease.

The Kidney governs birth, growth, and development
One's whole life span is controlled by the Kidney Essence. For women, life is marked in 7-year cycles. For men, it's 8-year cycles. Here is an example using a woman's life cycle

0-7 years	Early childhood
7-14 years	Begin school, get permanent teeth (teeth are a surplus of bone which is controlled by the Kidney). You get 52 total teeth including baby teeth throughout life.
14-21 years	Menstruation commonly starts around age 14. Then there's all that fun teenage angst I hope to never have to go through again.
21-28 years	Best ages for pregnancy, with 28 being the peak. You couple up, get married/get a domestic partner. But for the healthiest offspring, don't get pregnant before the age of 21!
28-35 years	Raising kids, building your home life, starting a career
35-42 years	Building your career, hopefully getting those kids out of the house.
42-49 years	Schedule that midlife crisis. Essence is exhausting and menopause starts poking at you. This doesn't mean you are dying, just running out of stuff to pass on the kids and losing your vigor.

This is a very old theory and life spans have changed since then, but the basics are still true.

For best longevity, health care should be well established by age 28, which is when your energy drops. Qigong, dietary therapy, herbal therapy can all help to build good acquired Essence so that you don't have to tap into the pre-heaven Essence your mom and dad gave you. It is never too late to expand, strengthen, and conserve that pre-heaven Essence! You only get one dose of that, so treat it well and make it last.

(Note: a lot of practitioners will tell you you only get so much and when you spend it you're out. But Daoist masters will tell you that you can truly replenish your pre-heaven Essence by practicing Qigong.)

Dr. Qianzhi Wu, my Foundations professor, and an awesome practitioner, recommends Bone Soup to help with this preservation and build up the Kidneys. I know this has become extremely popular and you can buy it in Whole Foods, but this one is way better and less processed.

Here's his recipe:

Dr. Wu's Bone Soup/Broth
- Use clean bone (any kind). Cut and boil it for 2-3 minutes (it tastes awful if you don't), then discard the water…or give it to the dog. Mine loved that.
- In a clean pot, add…
    - Water
    - The clean bone from the previous step
    - 3 pieces of ginger
    - 5 pieces of scallion
    - Salt
- Simmer for 6-8 hours.
  Add in beans, tofu, vegetables, etc toward the end of the cooking cycle so that they do not cook into mush. I mean, if you feel like you need to "hearty" it up.

When the soup is done, consume. Eat the bone too if it got soft enough while cooking.

Kidney governs Reproduction
The Kidney has lots more functions in Chinese medicine than it does in western medicine. How does it govern reproduction? It stores Essence (also known as Tian Kui). This is similar to the concepts of estrogen and testosterone hormones. Tian Kui controls maturation of the reproductive organs as well as menstruation.

If hormones are in excess, the Liver is affected. The result is often emotion swings and PMS. If the hormones are deficient, the Kidney is affected. This can result in irregular cycles, amennhorea, and scanty periods. Always care for the Kidney during menstruation and menopause, but especially in menopause.

Age 49-51 is the common age range for onset of menopause. Menopausal women typically suffer from poor sleep, hot flashes, emotional swings, and vaginal dryness/atrophy. All of these are symptoms of Kidney Yin Deficiency.

The Kidneys produce Marrow, fill up the Brain, and govern the Bones.

What is marrow? Isn't that the goo inside your bones? From a biomedical perspective, yes. But in Chinese medicine it is much more.

Marrow is Yin and fluid-like and there are three types.

Type of Marrow	What happens when that's not healthy
Bone Marrow	Weak knee joints are the result of a weakened Kidney essence. Cartilage too is related to the Kidney essence. Joint pain, articular degeneration, herniation of discs, bone spurs, and sciatica can all result
Spinal Marrow	When not in balance or depleted, herniation of discs, sciatic pain
Brain Marrow	The Brain stores marrow and is called the "Sea of Marrow." Alzheimer's, dementia, and bone loss are all due to the exhaustion of Kidney essence which results in not enough marrow to fill the brain or bones.

The Kidney meridian connects to the Brain when it connects to and enters the spinal column. When Kidney connects to the spine it also links to the Du channel, an extraordinary channel with its own points, which has very strong connections to the Brain and brain functions.

Look back at the Heart notes and you will see reference to the Kidneys controlling long term memory and the heart controlling short term memory. For best intelligence, harmonize the Heart and Kidney.

During infancy the forehead fontanelles are open, there are no teeth and no knee caps. If you can strengthen the Kidneys you strengthen these areas. It is said that the Tibetan form of ritual prayer in which they pray, kneel on the knees, and touch the forehead to the ground strengthens the Kidneys. For bone fractures, tonify the Kidneys to speed healing – use acupuncture and herbal therapies as well as bone soup. (See recipe above)

Kidney governs water

Body Fluids are stored in the Bladder, but they are not considered urine until they are excreted. While they are in the Bladder they are steamed by the Kidney Yang and can be recycled back to the Lung. The Lung can then disperse them further to the skin for skin moisture. If you exercise in the morning before you urinate you won't have to pee afterwards (or not as much) because the liquid will have been reclaimed by the body! And yes, I know biomed denies that this can happen. Whatev. I've tried it and it worked. Thanks, Dr. Wu.

The Kidney governs the water of the body – the Kidney Qi governs the opening and closing of the Urine Bladder. While the Bladder opening is closed, the fluids remain. *All* urination problems are due to Kidney dysfunction. Difficult urination, retention of urine, incontinence, and dribbling all fall under this umbrella. Treat the Kidney and you will treat the root of the problem.

Kidney controls reception of Qi

We've talked about this before. There are three sources of Qi:
- **Da Qi**
  Da means big. You have to have the source constantly or

you die. That source is air, and yeah, that makes this pretty big! Da qi comes from the Lungs and is generated in the Upper Jiao
- **Gu Qi**
  Gu Qi comes from food and drink. It's produced in the Middle Jiao by the Spleen and Stomach.
- **Primary Qi**
  Primary Qi comes from the Kidney in the Lower Jiao.

But even the breath and Da Qi are rooted by the Kidney. The Kidneys, when they are working well, will grasp and hold the breath long enough for Qi to be extracted from it. Ren 4 and 6 are points below the umbilicus on the midline of the body. They are where the Lower Dantian is seated. This area is part of the Kidney energy and are about where the breath is rooted by the Kidneys. These points should never be sedated, as they are the *seat* of this holding function. This is the root of the body, the Sea of Qi. When a patient has asthma, bronchitis, or emphysema, tonify the Kidney Qi and the breath will deepen.

For chronic cases treat the Kidney, for acute cases (active asthma attack, i.e.), treat the Lung.

The Lungs *govern* the Breath
The Kidneys *root* the Breath.

Kidney opens to the ears

Kidney Essence can be monitored by the teeth, hair and ears.
- Teeth
  Problems with teeth (loose teeth, teeth that acquire cavities easily, teeth that break easily, etc.) can be due to weak Kidney Essence.

- Hair
  Loss of hair, hair that grays way to early, fragile or thin hair can be the result of poor Kidney Essence.

- Ears
  Long earlobes reflect a constitution geared toward longevity. Ringing in the ears can be due to Kidney Essence deficiency. For deafness and tinnitus from old age, tonify Kidney.

  Have you ever noticed that the shape of the ears looks an awful lot like the shape of the kidneys? That's called the 'doctrine of signatures' – that which looks like a thing is related to a thing. Brains look like walnuts and can actually help brain function. Kidney beans look like kidneys and are good for the too. Ears look like kidneys and reflect the health or disease of the Kidney.

Kidney manifests on the hair

Hair is a surplus of Blood while teeth are a surplus of Bone. Hair loss and alopecia are due to Kidney Essence Deficiency. Dryness and weakness of the hair can be due to Liver Blood deficiency or Kidney weakness.

Kidney opens the two lower orifices (anus, urethra/vagina)

The anal opening is controlled by the Kidney. Chronic constipation/diarrhea is a Kidney related problem.

- Early morning diarrhea (between 5am and 7am)
  This is also called "cock's crow diarrhea" in Chinese medical literature. When the Kidney Yang is deficient one of the signs/symptoms is early morning diarrhea. It can also express as excessive vaginal discharge.

- Kidney Yin deficiency can express as nocturnal emissions in men, with or without dreams that accompany them.

- Kidney Qi deficiency can result in incontinence of either urine or stool.

Kidney houses willpower

If one lacks motivation and/or has feelings of hopelessness, tonify the Kidney. Use moxibustion techniques at the level of L2 on the spine, which is the Du 4 point, to encourage Kidney Qi to move upward.

The Kidneys are the Gate of Vitality or Ming Men

About 1800 years ago the *Difficult Questions* work was published. These consisted of 81 questions and answers. This work established that the Kidney is two organs: left is the organ itself while the right was described as the Ming Men. In the 13th Century Dr. Zhao Xian Ke said no, both are organs; the Ming Men is *between* the Kidneys. Primary Qi is in this area.

Within the Kidney is a fluid-like essence. Dr. Zhong Jingyue said the left Kidney is the home of the Kidney yin while the right Kidney is the home of the Kidney yang. If a Kidney is removed, one will have deficiency accordingly.

The Ming Men has the following functions. Most schools don't have you memorize these at this stage but you definitely want to pay attention to this, especially in some of your later education. When you gets to herbs you'll hear about a few that 'return the fire to its source.' This refers to tonifying the Ming Men.

- Root of Primary Qi
- Source of Fire for *all* internal organs
- Warms the Lower Jiao and Urinary Bladder
- Warms the Spleen and Stomach, assisting in digestion. Food will not ripen/rot without it!
- Harmonizes sexual function, warming semen and uterus.
- Assists Kidney function of the reception of Qi
- Assists the Heart's function of housing the Shen/Mind.
-

Dreams

Not a function exactly, but something you need to know: if one dreams of swimming after a shipwreck it reflects a desire for water and swimming in general – and reflects Kidney deficiency.

Sayings from various Chinese medical texts

- The Kidneys have no excess!
  Never sedate them. Never. Even when you learn Five Element theory and you see "sedate the Kidneys." Don't do it. Urinary Bladder, yes, but not the Kidney.

- Women have Liver as the most important organ while men have Kidney as the most important organ. Practice celibacy – about 100 days per year – in order to preserve Kidney essence.

- The Kidney does not like Dryness
  It stores fluid-like Essence and needs moisture.

FUNCTIONS OF THE URINARY BLADDER

1. Receive and store Body Fluids
   (*not urine!* Urine isn't urine until it's exiting from the body. Until then it's still "body fluid" and TCM says the body can reabsorb the moisture when it's still in the Bladder.)

2. Discharge urine with the help of the Kidney
   Kidney Qi/Yang governs the transformation. Normal fluids become turbid until the Kidney transforms them. The Kidney controls the opening and closing of the Bladder. When closed the Kidney Yang steams the fluid upward to the Lung. When open, the Bladder discharges, producing urine. This controls the water metabolism of the body.

3. Body Fluids plus accumulated Dampness and Heat in the Bladder can produce stones. Remove the damp and heat to treat stones.

> The Kidney *suffers no excess*,
> but the Urinary Bladder is *prone to excess*

About the Author

Cat Calhoun is a licensed acupuncture practitioner in the State of Texas and soon to be in the State of Florida as well. She attended AOMA Graduate School of Integrative Medicine, earning a Masters degree in Acupuncture and Oriental Medicine. She is passionate about teaching, both formally and informally. Cat has single-handedly created and managed CatsTCMNotes.com since 2008, dispensing notes and clinical pearls to students and practitioners for the past 11 years. She is also passionate about learning, and is currently in love with Master Tung's Acupuncture system.

This book, *Chinese Medicine 101: Start with the foundations*, has a companion book for the 2nd half of your Foundational education in Chinese medicine. Look for it Amazon: *Chinese Medicine 102: Complete your foundations*. Both of these books are vital for framing your understanding of the philosophy and basic understanding of Chinese medicine.

www.ingramcontent.com/pod-product-compliance
Lightning Source LLC
Chambersburg PA
CBHW021829170526
45157CB00007B/2728